Praise for *Own Your*

"This powerful, inspiring, and luscious book is an [...]
all women, no matter what age, color, size, or am[...]
and profound skill, Latham leads us through the process of shedding the
inauthentic self and cultivating the radiant being within, the woman inside just
waiting to be born. *Own Your Glow* is an essential primer for women looking to
transform, thrive, and take up all the space in this world that they deserve. Full
of affirmations, recipes (for smoothies and body butter!), and sage, scientifically
sound advice from around the world, this book is a primal call for women to slay
the demons within and emerge victorious and . . . *glowing*."

— Rebecca Walker, feminist and *New York Times* best-selling author

"Deep, wise, inspiring, and fun, Latham is *your* shaman for achieving the
seemingly impossible: putting yourself first and navigating the occasional
chaos and challenges of being female with joy and style."

— Wednesday Martin, Ph.D., #1 *New York Times* best-selling author
of *Primates of Park Avenue*

"*Own Your Glow* is just the indulgent trip inward we need to dust off the
cobwebs and embody the luminous royalty we can actually become, and
enjoy if we dare. I want to glow like Latham, so I'm going for it. Join in!"

— Tara Stiles, founder of Strala and author of *Guiding Strala*

"The beautiful words in *Own Your Glow* inspire me to overcome my biggest challenges
and to never hold back from expressing my true self. I am so thankful for strong,
courageous, and graceful mama leaders like Latham who are changing the world!"

— Vani Hari, founder of Food Babe and *New York Times* best-selling author
of *The Food Babe Way*

"Every time I see Latham, I instantly feel better. Her energy is calming but powerful.
She exudes the confidence to walk with queens but also accessibility and common
touch. I always wished she'd bottle that. And, thankfully, she just did. Lucky us."

— Nicole Lapin, finance expert, TV personality,
and *New York Times* best-selling author of *Rich Bitch*

"Latham is everything to me, a real-life unicorn. In *Own Your Glow*,
she dishes her priceless wisdom and makes it accessible for everyone.
I'm so glad we all get a taste of her magic."

— Luvvie Ajayi, *New York Times* best-selling author of *I'm Judging You*

"Latham has birthed a profound manifesto of how to live life so we can embody
the radiance and brilliance of who we truly are. This is a woman who teaches by
example and walks her talk—and it is out of her immense generous heart and spirit
that this book was born, pouring out wisdoms and sacred practical principles to
make our everyday lives glow with the vibrancy of the gift of simply being alive!"

— Agapi Stassinopoulos, author of *Wake Up to the Joy of You*

"In *Own Your Glow*, Latham Thomas shatters the glass ceiling and outlines the
pathway of true success. For generations, feminine power has been suppressed; this
book is the pathway to reclaim your feminine and discover your inner power. Bravo."

— Mastin Kipp, best-selling author of *Daily Love*

"It's divine time for this guide, for sister-women everywhere who are committed to self-care and remaining centered in these noisy times. Thomas ignites the feminine energy within us all, and the resulting formula within the pages of this gift are invaluable, accessible, and essential for honing our spiritual and professional selves."

— Raquel Cepeda, filmmaker and author of *Bird of Paradise*

"*Own Your Glow* unlocks the secret to true style. It starts from the inside out, and Latham has found a way to guide you in tapping into your inner confidence that one needs to be captivating and convincing and to conquer some of life's biggest obstacles. Style is more than a fashionable outfit you put on. It's your voice, a strong sense of awareness. This book simply will help you glow up in style."

— June Ambrose, celebrity stylist and designer, author of *Effortless Style*

"Glow on. This book will allow you to do just that. Through your good days and even your bad days, glow maven Latham Thomas breaks down the anatomy of our glow and provides us with the keys to unlock that power in each of us. Here's a tip—read it with Post-it notes and highlighters. You will want to revisit it time (and time) again."

— Lisa Price, founder of Carol's Daughter

"It is not often when you find people who enter your life that bring with them a light that shines so bright that you have to pause and ask yourself, *How I am so lucky to have this energy transcend into my world?* That light . . . Latham Thomas. That book . . . *Own Your Glow*. I am looking forward to the spiritual and inspirational journey Latham will take us on to discover and awaken the inner beauty and strength we as women all have inside of us. I am certain it will be thought-provoking, self-awakening, and empowering on so many levels. Life is about leaving old chapters behind as building blocks and discovering the new. I am sure this book will open that new chapter and take your story, your journey, to the top of the bestsellers list. Can't wait!"

— Kimberley Hatchett, wife, mother, mentor, and financial wizard

"Latham Thomas has written a must-read for all women! An empowering road map to help us understand, give us the tools we need to embrace our feminine power, and remind us that the only way to live is to claim our passion, inspiration, creativity, and magic. Latham Thomas gives us permission to own our glow and fully express ourselves as powerful, vulnerable, and empathetic beings, who will always have the courage to stand in purpose. If there's one book *every* woman should read this year, it's *Own Your Glow*! We promise you, it will transform you and your life."

— Antoinette Clarke, Vice President of Branded Entertainment and Media Innovation, CBS, and Tricia Clarke-Stone, co-founder and CEO of Narrative

"*Own Your Glow* is an uplifting and soulful guide to living your best life. As a career mom about to conceive my second child, I needed Latham's words of rebirth to start a new chapter in my business and motherhood journey."

— Pauline Malcolm, business executive at Disney

"'Go, go, go, do, do, do! Superwoman, be ten times better. Strong black woman . . .' all of this messaging hit me out of the womb and was immediately modeled by other 'strong black women.' After swimming in a sea of ambition, I have often found myself rudderless in a time when I know my source of strength comes from within, from being still, from self-care, and from slowing down . . . glow maven bridges that awareness to the next appointed action of self-care . . . because for some of us, we need to be spoon-fed how to care for ourselves when our autopilot is, 'I'm fine.'"

— Mara Brock Akil, creator and showrunner of *Girlfriends*, *The Game*, and *Being Mary Jane*

"*Own Your Glow* is packed with practical wisdom on how to shine as you've always been meant to. From cultivating inner peace to discovering your life's true purpose to joyfully unleashing your own personal style, Latham Thomas guides you step by step along the fulfilling path to your 'glow zone.'"

— Sarah Jones, Tony Award–winning performer and writer

"A timely book for all women looking to really thrive in life! Written with passion and insight, this is the type of workbook I share with my clients and friends who are seeking more but aren't sure how to accomplish filling that inner void and are overwhelmed with current quick fixes. All too often I think of the quote, 'drowning in information but starving for knowledge.' Latham's wisdom combined with her grasp on a multifaceted approach to really finding one's path through spirit and honoring one's feminine essence is unparalleled. Blessed are the future generations of wise and wonderful women to have such resources."

— Claire Fountain, founder of Trill Yoga

"Latham Thomas is one of those very rare souls you meet in life who truly exemplifies pure love and energy. Now she's written a beautiful and generous book that shares her gift with women all over the world to unlock your full potential and live a genuine life where the universe conspires to help you and those around you experience your glow. I highly recommend anyone to experience infinite love through this book."

— Shauna Mei, founder of AHAlife

"Being a wife and mother while balancing your career requires a lot of preparation, and often as women we prep everything except for ourselves! Latham reminds us of the importance of mentally preparing yourself on a regular basis, while owning your *glow* in order to restore your drive and confidence. This book is a must-read for all women, as it walks us through the importance of knowing our strengths and maintaining our spirituality."

— Valeisha Butterfield Jones, co-founder and CEO of WEEN

"Goddess glow! Sister Latham offers us the soul food that we need, and it is as poetic as it is nourishing. Such a lovely reminder of the need to honor the divinity within ourselves and each other."

— Joy Bryant, actress and founder of Basic Terrain

"*Own Your Glow* is a treasure trove of tools catalysts, caregivers, and creators need to fortify their minds, bodies, and souls to rise to the occasion in fast-paced and sometimes turbulent times. It offers the perfect mix of spiritual pragmatism and visionary wisdom seekers need to trust their intuition and transform their lives through thoughtful and empowered practice. Latham inspires readers to claim their power and honor their stories with a strong and nurturing voice. Her guidance prepares you to turn up the volume on those truths that were in hiding or existed as mere whispers before. Get ready for the alchemy it creates inside to radiate externally."

— Jamia Wilson, feminist, movement builder, and storyteller

"A compelling ride of healing words that guides your heart, rattles your soul, and pulls your glow from within. *Own Your Glow* is essential and actionable. A must-read, a blueprint, *an art of healing*."

— Iesha Reed, director of brand communications, Swarovski

"Latham is not only an authority for me but an inspiration.
In a world that's moving at the speed of light, sometimes I feel like I'm
sitting in the dark. Latham has the ability to draw open the curtains and
let the sunshine back into my spirit where I can truly see who I am. Simply put,
Latham gives me the courage to have vulnerability in doing the unthinkable: really
seeing myself and owning my glow at a pace that I understand. *Own Your Glow*
has the power to transition your inner light outward, and gives you permission to
be exactly who you are in all your glory. Latham never fails to remind me of my
worth, and to have my own back against all the noise of the world."

— Tina Wells, CEO and founder of Buzz Marketing Group

"In an ever-fast-moving world that stretches the limits of 'having it all,' Latham
Thomas reminds us that we should have no guilt in exploring what energizes us
and deciding to live for us, not just for the world. Latham shows that embracing the
freedom to explore and define a personal vision and translating this into passion-
filled action are the key steps to living a confidence-filled and glow-full life."

— Morin Oluwole, head of Luxury, Facebook

"Being uniquely yourself is a blessing and responsibility and Latham
leads readers to take, discover, embrace, and take charge
of their unique gifts and imprint the world with their magic."

— Bozoma Saint John, global business executive

"*In Own Your Glow*, Latham reminds us that we are the designers of our
own lives and to inject personal style and personality into everything we touch.
This book is a must-read for anyone wanting to tap into that inner glow."

— Danielle Snyder and Jodie Snyder Morel, co-founders of DANNIJO

"Latham Thomas studies history, language, science, anatomy, and ancient rituals
for her practice. Whether she's conducting workshops, writing a life-changing
book like *Own Your Glow,* or guiding a birth, Latham arrives with both humility and
great authority. She always makes space for others to empower themselves and to
learn more about themselves, each other, and the interconnectedness of it all."

— dream hampton, writer, filmmaker, and activist

"There is no perfect life, but there is your better one! *Own Your Glow*
is packed with doable tips and tools to help each of us navigate our better path.
Read, gift, and enjoy your better results!"

— Ashley Koff RD, founder of The Better Nutrition Program

ALSO BY LATHAM THOMAS

Mama Glow: A Hip Guide to Your Fabulous Abundant Pregnancy

The above is available at your local bookstore or may be ordered by visiting:

Hay House USA: www.hayhouse.com®
Hay House Australia: www.hayhouse.com.au
Hay House UK: www.hayhouse.co.uk
Hay House India: www.hayhouse.co.in

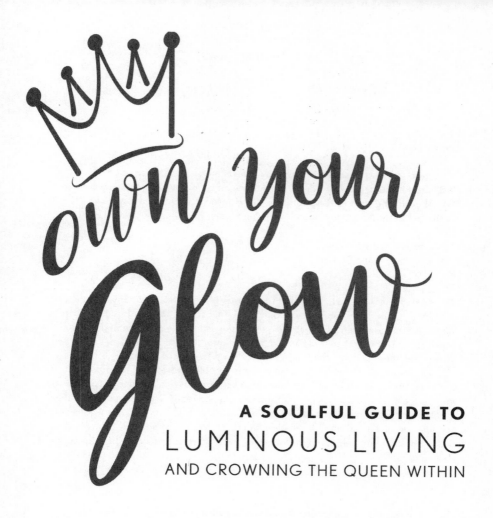

own your glow

A SOULFUL GUIDE TO
LUMINOUS LIVING
AND CROWNING THE QUEEN WITHIN

LATHAM THOMAS

HAY HOUSE, INC.
Carlsbad, California • New York City
London • Sydney • New Delhi

Published in the United States by: Hay House, Inc.: www.hayhouse.com®
Published in Australia by: Hay House Australia Pty. Ltd.: www.hayhouse.com.au
Published in the United Kingdom by: Hay House UK, Ltd.: www.hayhouse.co.uk
Published in India by: Hay House Publishers India: www.hayhouse.co.in

Cover design: Cara Budner
Interior design: Riann Bender

Cataloging-in-Publication Data is on file with the Library of Congress

Tradepaper ISBN: 978-1-4019-3923-6
E-book ISBN: 978-1-4019-4951-8
Audiobook ISBN: 978-1-4019-5741-4

10 9 8 7 6 5 4 3 2
1st edition, September 2017
2nd edition, June 2020

Printed in the United States of America

SALUTATION

Saluting the women of the world . . . The womb of the world. The creative matrix. . . . The ephemeral and the everlasting. . . . The dark, damp, and divine . . . The moody moon. . . . The goddess within and the priestess showing out . . . Saluting the cosmic dance of embodied Shakti undulating . . . Waves, water, womb. The future is, always, and forever shall be female. Woman is the beginning and within her lies a universe. Her ornate topography is sacred. Her hips are holy. Saluting her strength and bowing to her vulnerability. She is complex, complicated, compassionate, curious, cultivated. . . . She is inclusive, supportive, loving, gentle (but don't cross her), and kind. She is badass, breaking rules, blazing trails, and forging bonds. Spirit guide, big mama, boss lady, activist. She unites everyone. She uplifts. She is the crux of the community. She is a leader . . . The leader . . . The mother. Mama. Pregnant with promise. Womb ignited. Love coursing through her bosom. The future suckling at her breast. Slaying the agenda barefoot and in high heels, from bedroom to boardroom, from home to office, from city to countryside. May we reclaim the sanctity of our bodies. The world is spawned within each of us. Saluting those living in bondage (may we continue the fight for you), break the mold and stand firmly in our power to be a force for change. And to those thriving in liberation and using their glow power to be a force for good in this world (to whom much is given, much is expected), may we shine together as one, as WOMEN. May you be supported and guided by the light. This work is channeled from my soul, birthed through my fingertips onto these here pages, and dedicated to each of you . . .

One love,

Latham

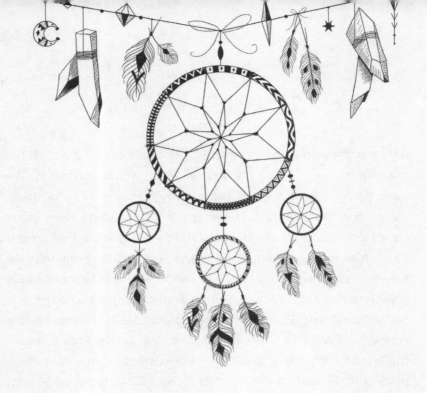

"*All that we are is the result of
what we have thought.*"

- Buddha

CONTENTS

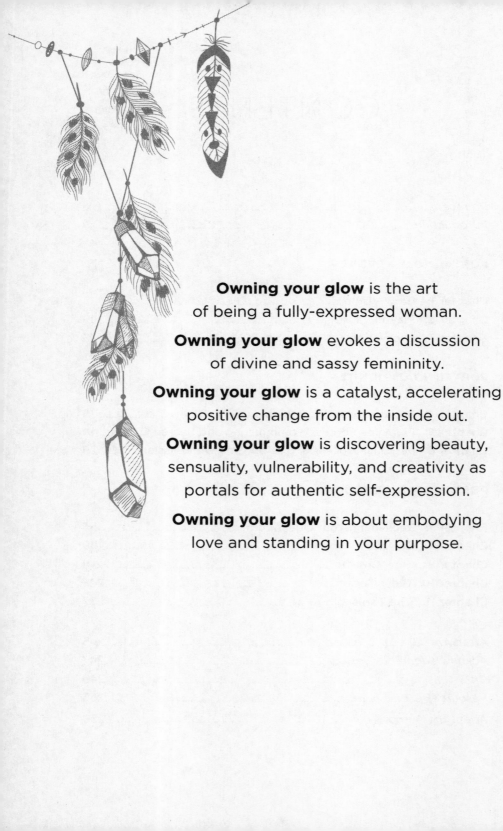

Owning your glow is the art
of being a fully-expressed woman.

Owning your glow evokes a discussion
of divine and sassy femininity.

Owning your glow is a catalyst, accelerating
positive change from the inside out.

Owning your glow is discovering beauty,
sensuality, vulnerability, and creativity as
portals for authentic self-expression.

Owning your glow is about embodying
love and standing in your purpose.

PREFACE

When I was little, I loved to play outside barefoot, to collect feathers and rocks, to spin in circles and lie in the grass, gazing up at the sky. Mother Nature recognized my potency, and I was fascinated with her rhythms. Blooming flowers stood tall in my presence, and oak trees told me secrets. I would chase butterflies and rainbows and jump-rope lightly so as not to disturb the earthworms. The ambient landscape was my playground, and it was expansive with possibility. When I was little, I thought the "twinkle in my eye" meant there was an actual star in my eye looking back at another star up high, gazing in wonder and admiration of its own reflection. The moon followed my every move at dusk, and the sun rose for my benefit at dawn. I believed I was made of stardust.

When I grew older, I learned about nebulae, which often appear like the iris of one's eye. They are interstellar nurseries for baby stars, planets, star systems, and galaxies. Their gigantic collections of space particles and gases spin furiously, resulting in creation vibration, giving shape to the expanding universe. Scientists say that about a teaspoon of the spinning gas and cosmic matter that made up the first stars in the galaxy lives within each of us today. So, we really are made of stardust after all!

That divine dance of cosmic energies swirling within each of us combines with our unique femininity to produce our creative edge, a force that awakens and amplifies the ability to draw unto ourselves what we most desire—to create the life we want, with every dream, thought, and intention. We are alchemists. We have the ability to take what life has handed us and transform it into something new, something greater than even we could imagine. That innate creative force within all women—cosmic-creation vibration, that potent instinctual energy that awakens within us, plus fierce femininity—*that* is what I call glow power.

Welcome to the *glow*! This book is about taking that cosmic dance inward, aligning with your internal galaxy, and being attuned to your own divine glow. You are a walking miracle, a divine piece of work! There was none before you, and there will never be another you once you're gone. This is your time to touch everything in your midst with your divine light, to imprint the world with your unique brand of magic, and to recognize that divine light emanates from deep within us—from the darkness. We need to remember that darkness gives birth to all things manifest.

We as women have been taught to fear our power, our darkness, our mysterious pull. To be ashamed of the very things that make us uniquely ourselves. We are afraid of the dark; we associate it with what's bad. I remember learning in elementary school science class that *black is the absence of light*. Along the visible spectrum, white reflects light and is the presence of all colors, but black absorbs light and is the absence of color. That struck me, because science was negating what my soul knew—that blackness is the light of the world. It's in the darkness that we find immense power and grace. The dark, dank soil nourishes root systems and gives rise to plant life. In the darkness of the womb, new life is spun into being. The dark night sky allows us to dream at night. It is a whole and necessary part of the cosmic order; darkness is divine.

Owning Your Glow is about trailblazing in our darkness to ignite the light around us and reclaiming every aspect of ourselves in spirit and in flesh. We must collectively plant seeds of confidence and conviction and weed out the messages undermining our power, beauty, radiance, and resilience. I'm inviting you to celebrate the aspects of yourself that you may have turned away from long ago, the dark places you are afraid to go within yourself. Bring them into the light so you can become your most powerful self and lure anything you want into your path. I'm inviting you to your initiation.

There is an ethereal glow that is maintained when we are in constant reverence of the divine source of creative energy flowing through us. That is the glow I am talking about and what I want to illuminate in you as we journey through this book together. We all have glow power. That light inside of you is relentless. Everything it touches in its path is graced. Here we will explore key lifestyle practices to ignite that inner light and keep it sparked, to make us irresistible in the boardroom, in the bedroom, and in the mirror. If you're at a crossroads in your life right now—if you're ready to leave your job, ready to find your life's partner, or ready to make that baby— and if you are holding parts of yourself back out of fear, judgment, or self-doubt, then this journey is for you.

Think of this book as your complete guide to luminous living and stepping confidently into your grace. It's a recipe for uncovering and focusing on the life changes you seek, embracing your unique feminine edge, exploring your strengths, swan-diving into your passions, and indulging in radical self-care to create a *glow-rious* life. There is a sensual, textured, prescriptive, grown-ass-woman-ness that laces this book. It's a calling to all women to awaken the divine and tap into our power source. This book is an elixir, a formula for standing in your truth and using your feminine edge to design a life worthy of YOU.

GLOW, to me, is more than something you possess or carry within you; it is an actual vibration that you emanate. This guide is about finding your own creative edge, your sexy sauce, unabashedly crowning yourself, blossoming into leadership, nurturing your own nebula, and moving from the darkness into your explosive glow power that will light up the universe. If we can connect to that creative center—listen to it, feed it, nurture it—we can grow in ourselves something much bigger than our own journeys and offer it up to the world. When you transform, everything around you will, too.

Creating anything takes patience, courage, faith, and an ideal environment for growth. *Own Your Glow* will boost your creative process, your confidence, and your glow power as you birth the life of your dreams. What is it that makes you want to get up every day?

What inspires you? What makes you tick? What makes you lift your head with pride?

Here's to the twinkle in your eye, my dear Glow Gazer. I'm glad you're here, that you were guided to this book. Let's spark the light and grow your glow to its full potential.

LOVE AND LIGHT,

Latham Thomas

INTRODUCTION

You're ready to play big, be bold, and expand, but want someone to hold your hand, right? This book is set up in three sections, which I call portals, and it is a progressive journey—each chapter is best explored after the previous one, guiding you along the path of transformation and integration.

In the first portal, Evoke, we'll prepare. We'll identify what needs to change for you to live your best life, we'll clear out the space needed to make room for that which you want to call forth, and we'll explore how incorporating a spiritual practice into your life can ready you for the first step on your journey and each thereafter. Then, once we know what we wish to achieve, we'll light the fire in the Ignite portal and uncover how best to achieve your aim. We'll explore the feminine forces at play in your life, and we'll scratch the surface of your individual process—how you work best, your strengths, and your vulnerabilities. We'll learn to trust that process and prioritize your purpose, all while honoring the Universe's divine timing. Finally, to truly embody our glow power, we'll enter the Embody portal and reclaim our queendom through self-acceptance and self-care, even leaning into effective dietary and exercise practices so that we can emerge a beacon of glow power for those around us.

You may get excited and want to read ahead, but stay with me and move with the orderly flow of the book. I'm an avid cook, so I liken following this path to seasoning a stew or building a robust sauce. We always start with the base—the onions. They temper the oil and set the tone for the pungent flavor. The oil begins to sizzle; the onions sweat and turn translucent. We begin to layer, allowing garlic to infuse the oil, then adding bell peppers and celery. Next, the dry spices unleash their aroma and power into the fragrant mixture. We can't just place all the ingredients in the pan at once; it won't have the same effect or intensity of flavor. Like the ingredients of a sauce, each portal in this book unleashes certain lessons and allows you to peel back your own layers and get clear with yourself. The glow tips found within are not just inspirational but *aspirational* and actionable, guiding you to finding your own glow power and then dialing it up to full blast with extra help from some leading luminaries in the worlds of health, entertainment, beauty, fashion, spirituality, and personal growth, who provide their anecdotes and inspirational quotes.

Giving rise to the best iteration of yourself is at the center of your journey. Step into a soulful-fulfilling life of freedom, transcending self-destructive habits and creating a blueprint for a more gratifying, centered, productive, and bountiful way of living. This book is an offering, a refreshing antidote to the hustle-hard, make-it-happen mainstream culture and fosters patterns of slowing down, intentionality, and a practice of self-care, which I believe is paramount for personal growth. Are you ready to witness your life transform? Are you ready to tap into the vast queendom that lies within you? It's time to dive in and *Own Your Glow*.

"*Nobody can go back and start
a new beginning, but anyone can start
today and make a new ending.*"

- Maria Robinson,
author of *From Birth to One*

portal no. 1

EVOKE

|i′ vōk|

Verb: to bring or recall to the conscious mind.

From Latin *evocare*, "out of, from" + *vocare*, "to call."

To call forth

The Call

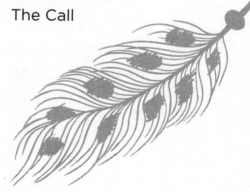

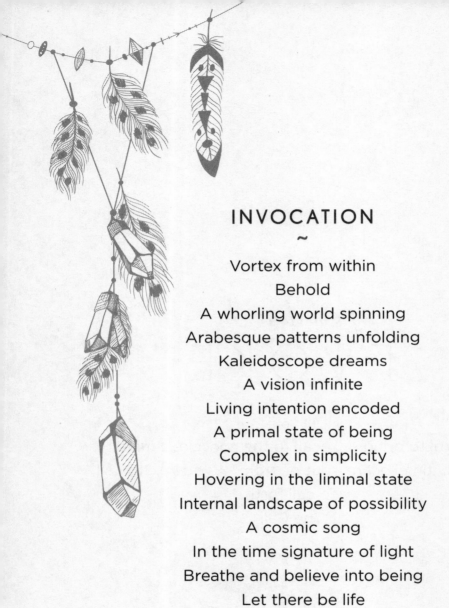

INVOCATION

~

Vortex from within
Behold
A whorling world spinning
Arabesque patterns unfolding
Kaleidoscope dreams
A vision infinite
Living intention encoded
A primal state of being
Complex in simplicity
Hovering in the liminal state
Internal landscape of possibility
A cosmic song
In the time signature of light
Breathe and believe into being
Let there be life

~

glow vision

"Your vision will become clear only when you look into your heart. Who looks outside, dreams. Who looks inside awakens."

~ CARL JUNG

*I*t's already a quarter past eight in the morning. She is rushing out the door, makeup bag in hand, and applying gloss as she simultaneously places her dramatic Tom Ford shades on to disguise the surprise: she's been up all night, and the bags under her eyes are in dire need of concealer. A multitasking machine—downloading important emails, replying to texts, and scrolling through Instagram, all while walking in four-inch heels down the block—her mind is already full of thoughts that aren't even her own. Anxiety takes over as she struggles to find a taxi during rush hour. She beats herself up for overeating the night before, snoozing, oversleeping, and subsequently skipping out on her torture time at the gym. If only she had been awake on time, she wouldn't be feeling disheveled and scattered. The guilt settles in. Feeling the pressure of the day, she starts off with shallow constrictive breathing that leaves her with subpar energy. Coffee will fix that; she indulges in three cups without even noticing.

She works ferociously at building a career for herself in a field that she isn't passionate about. She'd started with a moderate spark of interest and decided to pursue it because it paid well. It pleased her overbearing parents. Student loans are real, so she didn't have a choice. Or did she? She is making a decent living, but is it the life that was intended for her? She's too busy, caught up in the hustle, to hear the whispers of her soul, let alone acknowledge them. Does this sound like someone you know? Does this sound like you?

We all know an alpha woman, one who is doing it all. Driven, focused, "making it happen," striving—but not necessarily thriving—her way to the top of her game. The woman who sacrifices her own dreams so she can attain success is celebrated in our culture. One who is well-behaved, who says yes, who is an outputting machine able to outperform everyone else no matter what the circumstances, and she does it all in a pencil skirt or a pantsuit and with a smile. She might be single, an overworked mom doing it all, or a woman whose marriage to her work has been one of many factors leading to divorce. She is powerful beyond measure but lacking tether to her vulnerability. She is living a life that others would envy on the outside, but within, she is longing for connection, an anchor to something deeper. She wants to expand beyond the confines of the path that was set before her, one that outlines her destiny as others see it. She wants to awaken the dormant parts of herself, shake her past, and become new. She wants to become a woman living her dreams, standing fully in her *glow power,* and defining an arc of success and spiritual fitness on her own terms.

Are you ready to awaken to your dream? Are you ready to rise up to your greatness? Are you prepared to raise your own personal bar? If you answered a big YES to all three of those questions, then you are in for a beautiful and soulful ride, my friend. In this book we embrace the themes of boldness, confidence, and risk. And it was inspired by what I see as a lack of women embracing their unique feminine advantage. Women are the most powerful resource on the planet, and when we access, utilize, and harness what I call our *glow power*—our intuition and creative feminine edge—we can impact every aspect of our lives for the better, whether career, finances, love and relationships, spiritual life, body, or exercise. Go with your inner fire and be bold. Sometimes you have to put on your super heroine suit even when you can't yet fly. You have to be able to see yourself and envision what is possible and have hope even beyond that. You have to be willing to stand up for yourself and your potential and own your glow. Now the question is, who are you, really? What are you passionate about? What is missing that's keeping you from living your best life? The first step to embracing your glow lies in answering those questions.

First we need to define a seed goal, one we'll reach for throughout this journey. A seed is encoded with potent information and is suspended in animation until it is planted. A seed goal is a dense goal that we nurture through our intentions and actions, giving rise to a potent version of ourselves in the process. As women, we have an innate desire and need to create. When we merge our creative energy with love, we find passion taking us to new heights. It keeps us in a place of wonder. You may have started on your path toward success with someone else's dreams hovering over you; perhaps your parents had ideas of what and who you should become. That parental or societal vision may have molded your childhood activities, shaped your goals, and dictated your aspirations. But you've outgrown your kitten heels and stepped into your big-girl stilettos, and the world is much different than you imagined. And on this journey, we're working to harness the divine creative force within us so we can bring that extension of ourselves to fruition. Our goal might be a promotion, a new career, a new relationship, a *better* version of our current relationship, a healthier body/lifestyle, starting a family, or a more relaxed/organized existence.

Have you ever been in that place where suddenly nothing you've been doing makes sense and you just don't have the pep-in-your-step for your current job or relationship? You are afraid to explore the unknown, but you find it intriguing. You are here to find your passion and express yourself through that passion, to make a mark on the world and make a difference. Each of us has a mandate at birth, and not one of us was sent here without the capacity to achieve it. When you find something that excites you, something that makes you rethink your footsteps and feels like play, then you've tapped into your glow, a force within you that will guide you toward your wildest dreams.

Let's work together to uncover what it is you're striving for or what's percolating deep within you. You might sense or already know that something's amiss but can't figure out what exactly to do about it. In that case, I will help you discover it in the chapter ahead. You may already have a seed goal in mind, and if so, you should use the next chapter as a way of focusing that deep desire. If you already know what your seed goal is, write it here, and we'll expand upon it. If you don't yet have a handle on it, consider this neutral, empty space, and we'll discover together what you'll fill it with.

Your Current Seed Goals at a Glance

Remember, this is meant to be a path of growth, so you don't need to dwell on this. If you have something on your heart and mind, write it down. On a separate piece of paper or in a notebook, write down a few goals. This list is not meant to be exhaustive but a short list of goals that you desire to achieve most.

Listening to the Whispers (Tuning In to Your GPS)

Have you ever made a decision that goes against your "gut feeling"? Usually you feel terrible afterward not having listened to those signals, because the outcome isn't aligned with what you desire at your core. It could be as simple as "something told me to take that back-road route," but you didn't listen and found your way to standstill traffic on your way to work. Or it could be as big as feeling that something isn't quite right with the deal memo you are about to sign for an opportunity that comes your way.

That guiding voice from within is what I call your "GPS"—your Glow Power System—and acknowledging it is an essential part of owning your glow. We all come programmed with this innate tuning system, and while we often turn down its volume, the signal always works. Your body will give you signals that align with what your spirit knows. It will tell you whether or not you are on the right path. It will tell you quite simply *yes* or *no*, good or bad, in any given situation. Our GPS works with our body to generate feelings that we should use to help inform our decisions. It guides us toward what is truest for us.

Everything in existence once started small, at seed level. Take your mind to a place outside of your comfort zone and dream *big*. Expand your consciousness around what you want to create. Sometimes it's not that we aren't creative enough but that we don't believe in our own creative capacity. We haven't been taught to cultivate it but instead to shut it off and filter bits of it through for convenience. Our heavy reliance on logic and rhetoric takes us out of the moments where the whispers are calling us. Instead, we have to allow ourselves to meander, to get out of our headspace and into the expansive space that awaits.

I've always been fascinated with butterflies, and I became enthralled with fireflies when I spent my summers on the East Coast as a little girl. It seems impossible to catch a butterfly or firefly at first. You're so focused on following its beauty, its light, that you end up wandering off into a different place. And when you look up, suddenly you realize you are in a new realm, among new scenery. A firefly might lead you deeper into the darkness of a forest on a warm summer's eve. A butterfly might take you on a journey to reach higher as it rides the wind on a sunny day. Your creative impulse is like the firefly or the butterfly. It can be evasive, but if you follow its flickering light and allow it to take you on a journey, you can catch it.

While we are working together, you will learn to cultivate an active listening to this internal wisdom and creativity through several methods. You will activate and tune in to your GPS by acknowledging your dreams (those you have while you sleep as well as those that come in times of wistful imagining in the daytime), by nurturing passionate and creative pursuits designed to relax you and open you up to divine inspiration, and by cutting out the ever-present noise of technology. You'll open yourself up to internal whispers that may in some cases become loud voices guiding you to what's next. Trusting that inner wisdom is essential for any woman who owns her glow. Tapping into your GPS in these ways will help you zero in on your mission. Continue to nourish it, and it will guide you as you travel on this journey. Your GPS is a gift. Use it to your advantage.

Night Vision

Close your eyes. What do you see when your eyes are shut? Some of us experience a heightened sense of sound around us when sight is taken away. But some of us *see* when our eyes are closed. We see what we have been focusing our imagination upon. We see what brings us delight, love, joy, excitement. I'm here to help you develop that night vision so you can navigate your dreams with keen direction.

I remember being a little child and daydreaming, doodling, and not being punished for it. I would envision my future and talk in lofty speech and grandeur about who I was going to become. Nowadays, if a child doodles during class, she is considered unfocused and diagnosed with ADHD. If she thinks outside of the box, she is a misfit. If she dares to share her imaginative wisdom, she is swiftly put in her place. If employees daydream, they are guilty of compromising the productivity of the company, not celebrated for creative potency and fertile imagination. We don't value creative process in our culture today, yet we place tremendous value on the outcome of the creative process. We want all the results but don't want to put in the work required to achieve it. I find that peculiar.

To summon forth brilliance, you need to set the tone for it, make space for it. Creative solutions do not always come when you are deep in thought but when you are deep within. The voice that speaks to you when your eyes are closed—when you're off daydreaming, doodling, meditating, or even sleeping—is the voice of your intuition. That voice will guide you and help order your steps when you choose to listen.

Dream as Action

You are a creatrix; as God creates, so do you. You have the ability to bring forth new beings made in your image, new visions, dreams manifest. Dreaming is the language of the body. We are all spiritual beings, and for dreams to come to fruition, we must journey deep within ourself and learn to know our self and our body as the sacred vessel in which the seed of creativity grows. To experience any soul-ful shift, we must reframe our thinking and use different tools to achieve a different outcome.

Imagination is a powerful tool that can transform your body, your thoughts, and your future. In many ancient traditions, dreaming has been an integral part of rituals, mysteries, healings, and procre-ation. Creation and transformative stories all begin with a vision or dream. Your imagination is the secret to preparing your psyche and your body for the demands of your dream come to life. Tapping that imagination is about slowing down, stripping the pretenses, going within, really stirring up and evoking the dream powers to restore the creative act within you.

The belief that our bodies have nothing to do with our visions, hopes, aspirations, and fears has led to a deep ignorance of our psyche's power on the physical. Our psyche filters our view of real-ity through those very lenses. Our identity, as we move through the past, present, and future iterations of ourselves, arises from this field of images—visions involving bodily movements, sensations, and emotions of which we are barely aware.

Can we repattern our destiny by responding to and engaging with the rich landscape of our dreaming? I say yes! When we are asleep, when we are doodling and daydreaming, when we envision a goal, talk about our aspirations, or pursue an ambition—that is all dreaming in action. The right hemisphere of the brain is engag-ing in dreaming all the time; it's instantaneous and interactive. By responding to your dream images, you are given license to play. Your dreaming can become an instrument of your ambition, focus-ing your intention toward an aspiration. Responding to your dream images means quite simply becoming aware. Your self-inquiry and willingness to dive deep and learn more from your subconscious mind could be a pathway to cultivating the life you desire.

How to Dream

As children we were all very aware of our dreaming. When my son was small, he had a bad dream about a giant ladybug and insisted that it lived under his bed and he wouldn't sleep there. Every night I had to go under the bed and show him, "See? Nothing is here." The spooky dreams might shape a reality too—one that we aren't keen on but believe in nonetheless. As children, we also recall "good dreams" and seamlessly blend our subconscious fantasy into our waking life. This facility for seamlessly flowing between worlds was bred out of many of us but is necessary if we're to uncover our heart's truest desire, to reacquaint ourselves with the powerful childhood language of dreams. There are two ways to tap in. One, you can recall your nighttime dreams, or, two, you can tune your eyes inward to the vision field.

Think of a movie theater; your vision field is like a screen that displays what the mind projects. That may sound abstract, but it's in fact the simplest thing to do. Once you are aware of your dreaming, you're ready to become an active participant in your own mind/body experience. Your body will show you images of what it is experiencing, and you can communicate with it by responding in images, or visualizing. With the subconscious, your language of choice is always images. By dialoguing with your body, you become a partner in helping it meet its challenges and maximize performance.

Think of elite performance athletes. They train their bodies not just by doing, but by visually rehearsing the moves. A hurdler sees herself sprinting, rounding her spine, extending her leading leg, engaging her hamstring, hovering in space over the hurdle, floating her leading leg down, her cleat hitting lightly on the track while her hind leg makes a graceful exit over the hurdle, and she is off and sprinting until the next hurdle. When you learn to quiet your left brain momentarily and be fully involved in your dreaming, you will give birth to whatever is within you in a state of heightened awareness. Athletes call this "the zone," when they are one with mind, body, and spirit. I call it the glow zone. And when we are in this state, everything becomes effortless, automatic, and fluid.

You may not have any hurdles to visualize, but we can use the same technique to help discover our mission—the key is repetition. If you do it once and nothing happens, don't let that deter you. You can use imagery to create a clean slate so your mind is open and ready to receive the symbolism and messaging that may lead to your epiphany. For instance, if you're "searching for purpose," you might project in your vision field a staircase leading to an attic. You carefully climb up the stairs until you reach a very neat and organized attic full of filing boxes. And inside the boxes are memories and desires you've filed. Taking your time, you uncover each box and discover what has been waiting and lying dormant within you.

Every time you create images, you speak to your body. You create images in your night's dreams and your daydreams when you paint, sculpt, draw, or design a dress. You can communicate with the deepest recesses of your body through imagery. This tool can be powerful for healing past wounds, cultivating a vision, and actualizing your goals.

Where to Dream

Having a place to dream is not a luxury, it's a necessity. Your primary dream space may be your bedroom. It should be a relaxing, inviting space. The ancient Chinese art of Feng Shui states that warm, rich earth and skin hues such as terra cotta, copper, coral, cream, peach, tan, and cocoa create a cozy, welcoming atmosphere in the bedroom. Soft, natural colors like light blues, greens, and lavenders lend the bedroom a quiet, tranquil vibe and invite healing energy into the space.

The calming effect of an open, uncluttered space does wonders for your creativity. When your space is disorganized, so becomes your life. (I always say, "Messy bed, messy head.") When your room is organized—your nightstands are in order, clothes are neatly placed in drawers and closets—you create the ultimate space for dreams to flow. Keep some of your favorite essential oils or flower essences near your bedside and a journal and pen for fluid thoughts and *soul-scribing* upon waking up.

But your bedroom is not the only space where dreaming happens. Whether you work in a traditional office, cubicle, or co-working space, creating a beautiful space to work in can boost self-confidence and inspiration to breeze through your toughest projects. Make your workspace your own; infuse yourself into it.

You want the space to breathe yet still provide structure, allowing you to get work done while feeling whimsy and creative freedom at the same time. If you're in a monochromatic space, add an accent color through a bold chair or a patterned rug. Always keep fresh plants around so life is thriving in your workspace; fresh-cut seasonal flowers remind us that beauty is abundant and that we are deserving of it. Create a moment of reprieve, inhale deeply and breathe in the scent of your fresh flowers. I love a great desk lamp and images of inspiring women, plus a favorite quote or two to keep myself on track.

When working in public spaces in a freelance capacity, always bring some settling elements to contain your space within the public arena. Be mindful of the space you choose to settle into. Is it transient? Are there quiet areas where you can tuck away? Is there a window with access to a view or sunlight? Is it quiet? Do you meet nice people there? Is it clean and well kept? Do you feel good in this space? Choose your spaces wisely, as you will be marinating in the energy of that space while completing your tasks. Your favorite coffee mug, a notepad, or a seashell (which symbolizes fertility and creative force) are all things that can help you set the tone for dreams to flow.

Outside of your bedroom dreamspace and your work dreamspace, you need a joy dreamspace—an area where you go to practice what brings you joy as a pathway to the pursuit of your dreams. This place of pleasure is meant to evoke a sense of nurturing, beautiful aesthetics, and spiritual anchoring, as well as function. I had a client who designed a vacation home with the yoga room at the very top of the house, at its highest point. She wanted to be closer to the sky when practicing yoga and wanted to elevate the practice in her life. I am asking you to design your life around your dreams, weave them into your life through mindful integration. You don't need a yoga room, just a place where you go for fulfillment. That could be your bathtub, the spa, a beautiful library, your kitchen, a piano, your favorite patch of grass under an oak tree, the sandy shoreline at your favorite beach. Wherever it is, go there and dream.

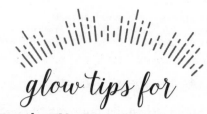

Sprucing Up Your Dreamspace

As we are products of our environment, consider your environment and how much time you spend there. Whether your space is super inspired or you feel in a rut, making changes to your dreamspace will open you up to your GPS and enhance your creative edge.

*Pillow **talk.*** One of the easiest ways to bring vitality into a space, particularly the living room or bedroom, is by swapping out pillows. Seasonal pillows allow you to bring punchy colors out for a spring twist and cozy winter colors and textures for the cooler months. I love bold patterns and bright colors. I even jazzed up my white dining chairs with colorful cushions. Don't be afraid to mix and match and experiment.

Deck the walls. Some people love white walls. I happen to love wallpaper and selected a textured wallpaper in my new apartment. I use art on the walls, as I am inspired by beauty. Enlarge your own photos and print them on canvas. Mix and match frames. Get your favorite quotes and place them on the walls for constant inspiration.

Go bold. Bold accessories can take a room from drab to artful and memorable. We often get shy, opting for safe and neutral choices, which can be beautiful—but embrace statement pieces that are colorful and sculptural; they make a huge impact on your space. I have a navy velvet sofa that anchors our living room and draws people in. Light up a room or desk with a fun lamp. Add flair to a room with colorful, patterned rugs and Moroccan cushions.

Happy hues. Paint can transform a room, no doubt. But it can take a lot to commit to a new color. As you choose the happiest hue for you, ask yourself:

- What colors make me happy?

- What hues do I choose to wear, and which make me feel my very best?

- What feeling am I aiming for?

If you're afraid to commit but need the change, use your colors sparingly and creatively by painting an accent wall or door. If you're finding it hard to choose, perhaps a wallpaper design might work as a great accent.

Surprise, surprise. Design choices are oftentimes unseen by those just passing through, hidden in a wallpapered closet or lined linen drawers. It's important to consider details and remind yourself that even the littlest things should be taken into consideration. My kitchen cabinets are lined with fabrics. It's a small detail that perhaps I only notice when I'm in the kitchen, reaching for one of my favorite mugs, but it makes a difference because it feels like a little unexpected surprise.

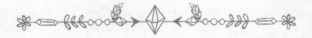

Dreams Are Free

Are there things you have always wanted to do or experience, share with the world, but you haven't seemed to make time for them? What are those things? As a single mother, I know this challenge of giving my dreams full attention very intimately. Is there a part of your life that has been put on hold while you wait for someone or some issue to be resolved before you can live out your dreams? What are these perceived obstacles?

Is there a part of your life where you do not feel emotionally fulfilled, where you feel a block in your pursuit? Close your eyes and get a sense of where that feeling lies in your body. It's easy to protect ourselves and come up with excuses for not pursuing our dreams, but I want you to share some examples of why you should actually go for it!

Dreams offer us freedom. Give yourself permission to start taking steps toward a part of your life that has not been fully expressed. Sometimes the bigger picture can be daunting when we are trying to figure out our first steps. What small steps can you take to prioritize your desires and set your intentions?

In her acclaimed bestseller *The Artist's Way*, Julia Cameron preaches about giving ourselves the permission to start fresh, from the beginning, to engage the beginner's mind. We always have the choice to end up with the pleasure of having pursued our dreams or the regret of keeping them on the back burner. Set an intention around a dream of yours.

Remembering Your Moonlight Dreams

What did you dream last night? Do you remember? Did you dream you were at the ocean, wading in her saline waters? Maybe you dreamed you were soaring through the night sky. Maybe you don't remember what you dreamed at all. We want to remember our moonlit dreams because they are a tool in our arsenal for self-discovery, creative problem solving, and attuning to our GPS.

Help yourself plug into your dreams by eliminating common inhibitors to restful sleep and dream recollection.

- **Create a bedtime ritual**. You should go to bed at roughly the same time every night, in the same place. Avoid sleeping in different areas of your home, like on the couch or in an armchair. Wind down by lighting an aromatic candle, taking a warm bath, cleansing your face, following with moisturizing your skin, turning off all electronic devices, taking a few minutes for mindfulness, and getting into bed.

- **Only sleep in your bed**. Don't check emails, talk on the phone, or eat in your bed. It's for three things only— sex, prayer, and sleep—and in that order.

- **Avoid watching TV late at night and falling asleep to programming**. Most infomercials come on late at night, and they enter our subconscious mind because we are most vulnerable then. If your favorite shows come on late, set a timer for your TV to turn off on its own so it doesn't remain on all night long.

- **Keep a vision journal.** Splurge on a pretty notebook and a nice pen to record the dreams you summon forth. Write the date, and leave the entry blank before going to bed. Leave the book open with your pen inside, setting your intention to remember your dream. As you drift off to sleep, remind yourself to remember. When you wake up, record everything you saw, heard, and felt in your dream, even if you think it doesn't make sense or doesn't seem important. (As you become wrapped up in your day, the dream will escape, so it's important to record what you remember before you even get out of bed.) Relax on your back to stimulate recall. Don't try to analyze; just allow yourself to feel what the dream is communicating. When you are ready, sit upright to record the dream.

- **Share your dreams.** Share your dreams out loud with your partner, mother, and/or friends.

- **Ask questions of your dreams.** After three weeks of recording your dreams and speaking them aloud, you are ready to ask questions of your dreams. You will use your thinking, conscious, rational mind to focus your dreaming mind. By focusing in, you narrow the field of stimuli and create a space for vision of your own interest. So, instead of your dreams happening *to* you, you are making space for your dreams to happen *for* you. Paying close attention to the imaginings of our dreamspace is just one method of opening ourselves up to the whispers of our GPS.

Dream Language: Mantras and Affirmations

Language has immense power. The words we use can aid in the agency of our dreams. We can use the potency of words to help reshape our habits, influence how we speak to ourselves, and to help impact our purpose and presence in the world. A mantra is a word, sacred sound, or phrase that directs energy toward concentration in meditation. A mantra is full of seed energy, or concentrated potential. An affirmation is a phrase that enhances positive thinking and encouragement. When you find yourself moving into negative thought patterns, use your mantras and affirmations to instantly lift your vibration and flip your perspective.

Rituals

Rituals amplify the magic in everyday moments. They are a series of actions performed with intention. They help to cultivate a deep sense of grounding and devotion toward oneself. Rituals can help crystallize your dreams, deepen your spiritual connection, and accelerate healing and self-discovery. We will explore practices that you can do alone as well as partnered. The rituals included here provide space for deep inquiry and integration, calling you to attune to your GPS.

Ritual Objects

Along our journey together, you will find that rituals call for some basic tools and objects. Having these things on hand will help prepare you for what lies ahead.

- Journal or notebook and pen
- Yoga mat and meditation cushion
- Found objects from Nature: feathers, seashells
- Crystals, stones, gems, and rocks
- Smudge sticks: *palo santo*, sage, incense cones, resins

- Bath salts, rose petals, dried flowers, herbs
- Art supplies: markers, paper, colored pencils, scissors, glue sticks
- Candles: devotional, scented, or beeswax or LED candles
- Sound: singing bowls, bells, music playlists

RITUAL
DREAM CATCHER!

Whatever your age now, we all start from a place of youth, innocence, and openness, with limitless vision and dreams. When you are young, there is no ceiling to your vision, no cap on the galaxy. It's infinite. And your possibility for greatness is infinite as well. Let's get back to that place of vast possibility. You're going to soul-scribe at the close of your day. Write down your biggest dreams, hopes, and desires on pieces of paper. On the other side, write an affirmation. Fold the paper and place it into a beautiful container—either one that you make or something you purchase. I call it a dream box. Mine looks like a jewelry box. Place this box near your bed where you sleep at night. Write down your hopes and dreams in the evening, and let them be the last thing you have on your mind before lights out. You will marinate in the energy of that dream as you relax and enter a sleep cycle. The Universe is living and in constant orbit, orchestrating miracles. We must be willing to soften and receive.

playful pause

*We don't stop playing because we grow old;
we grow old because we stop playing.*

~ George Bernard Shaw

Our culture is obsessed with productivity. Slowing down and making time to play allows us to transcend the monotony of our day-to-day lives and punctuate it with inspiration, often spawning new ideas and "aha moments." Play is important in all aspects of our lives, including creativity, work, and relationships. Europeans take long lunches with wine and conversation, followed by siesta or rest, and are still wildly productive. Maybe we should take heed! Taking a little break for ourselves helps slow down the brain waves, allowing us to transcend time and space momentarily while being captivated by something else, letting the whimsical little girl within come out to play.

Recreation = Re-Creation

Play is also an essential part of your GPS secret sauce. The word *recreation* comes from Latin's *recreare*, "to create again, renew." When we allow ourselves time for recreation, it offers us mental and spiritual consolation, allowing us to create again and make something new. Play helps us to transcend our normal beta-brain-wave thinking state and open up, take risks, stumble upon new strengths, and become aware of the areas where we need to grow. Play offers a safety net that allows us to dive into process without the pressures of performance associated with product or outcome. Play helps us to expand and be in the present moment of doing something that we love.

Give yourself permission to play every day. I don't mean break out the Monopoly board each time you want to have fun. It could be as simple as a game of fetch with your dog, hide-and-seek with your child, doodling on a napkin while waiting for your entrée at a restaurant, or a game of office ping-pong.

As an entrepreneur, I often get caught up in the hustle of running a business and only make time for meetings and client appointments, conference calls, and strategy sessions. The truth is, when I take time for myself to do something that takes my mind out of hustle mode, my most fruitful ideas are born. I have aha moments that in some cases contribute to problem solving or shaping my work in some meaningful way. Rather than creating a punitive model of work only and no play, integrate recreation into your daily routine. If you have interns or employees who work with you, it's also a great way to inspire them to generate new ideas. Give them time to play as well.

Google implemented a policy that allowed their engineers to spend 20 percent of their time working on anything they wanted. Products like AdSense and Gmail came from that free time. Plenty of other large tech companies have implemented their own takes on "20 percent time," including widely admired, innovative companies like Facebook, LinkedIn, and, reportedly, Apple. The core idea behind 20 percent time—that knowledge workers are most valuable when granted protected space in which to tinker and toy around—is a model now thriving in other industries today. At *The Huffington Post*, they not only have areas for recreation but nap rooms as well. Why not implement this principle into your workspace? If it stresses you out to think about playtime when you have so much to do, then think about it in these terms: "I will allocate one-fifth of my work time to myself and something that interests me."

We must shift the cultural perception we have that all work and no play is a good thing and that play is simply a waste of time and energy. Play is a healthy part of personal development and just as important for adults as it is for children. Melissa Goidal, chief revenue officer at Refinery29, the largest independent fashion and style website in the United States, says, "I don't have a job. I go to Refinery29 and get paid for it." In other words, she plays for a living.

Planned Play

Schedule your play. It sounds like the most neurotic thing, but trust me, it's necessary in a time when we are moving faster than ever before, with our calendars busting at the seams, leaving little to no personal time. When was the last time you took a trapeze lesson, went to a flamenco class, or sang the night away at karaoke? When you schedule every other part of your life, it doesn't leave much space for fun to weave its way in.

I love what I do. In my work, I get to go to Central Park in the early morning and do yoga with a client, attend a prenatal check up with a pregnant couple, grocery shop and cook for a new mom, attend the birth of a new baby, educate and mentor young doulas. Even still, as much joy as my work brings me, I carve out time to really relax, shut off, and chill. This is time for family, friends, and for me to spend alone. Play is an essential vitamin, so get your daily dose.

Playful Possibilities

If allocating space for play in your calendar has you rolling your eyes and sucking your teeth, then how about this mild approach to punctuating fun into your life on a daily basis? What playful plans should you integrate into your life? Fill in the blanks below, and you'll see for yourself what might spark an interest and be worthy of making space for.

I am having the most fun when I am _____

Time flies when I am _____

I wish I could do more _____

When I was little, I was always _____

My favorite childhood game was _____

My favorite pastimes have been _____

I'm really exceptional at _____

I'm fascinated by _____

The Passion Pursuit

When I am all work and no play, I am not the happiest me I can be. I am certainly not as productive and can be downright moody. Play is important. It's the primary focus of early-childhood development because it's fundamental and sparks creative vision. Incorporating creativity into your playtime can make recreation even more fruitful and passionate. It's the use of your imagination, employing original ideas, making new things, or making something out of nothing. To really have each of your days filled with abundant personal growth, you must engage in the processes that anchor you and allow you to expand and grow.

Passionate pursuits, even those not directly related to your ultimate goal or purpose, fuel the fire within. How can you infuse more creativity into your life? Just because you take an art class on Saturdays doesn't mean you're necessarily going to quit your job and become a visual artist. The art class allows your mind to still, to become quiet, open, and clear. In that sacred time you take to pursue your passion, you may stumble upon or have flickering moments of clarity about your life's journey.

Write down five things that you could do to make life more passionate and creative.

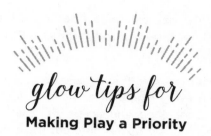

glow tips for
Making Play a Priority

Commit to a playful practice. The playful practice can be as small or as grand as you wish, but it must be something you will commit to on a regular basis. You can change it up, but commit to doing *something*. Assign yourself a few friends who will go on these play dates with you.

Get outside. There is energy in the atmosphere that you tap into when you breathe the fresh air and let the breeze whip through your hair and the sun kiss your skin. If you have access to a park or even the smallest patch of grass, take off your shoes and let your feet hit the soil. Uptake the charged energy of the soil through your feet and, whether you spend five minutes or five hours outside, your day will be changed for the better.

Tour your town. Take a leap and commit time on your calendar to exploring the very city you live in. Plan a staycation! You don't need a plane ticket or a hotel room, you just need a good pair of sneakers and a willingness to explore. This is a great idea for you if you have limited time but want to inject some spontaneous fun into your life.

Plan a Glow Getaway. The experience of travel fosters a sense of ingenuity. Packing a bag and heading off to a foreign land or even a place nearby provides a seat for inspiration and rejuvenation. We are awakened, removing the filter that we often wear at home. Go away, get lost, and find yourself. It's all about the journey and, in the end, the discovery. When we travel, we heighten a sensory experience and allow ourselves to be swept into a cauldron of languages, tastes, smells, colors, textures, architecture, customs, people, and fervent ideas. Whether you're doodling, daydreaming, or jet setting at 37,000 feet to your next destination, let your mind and heart wander together and carry you off to a place far away and deep within you.

Mix up your routine. If you shake up your perspective a bit, it can shift everything and turn a dull day into a playful one. If you are someone who sleeps in, wake up a little earlier to see the sunrise. Take a different route to work. Walk through the park on your way home and ride the swings. Get off the subway one stop earlier and take an alternate route. Press pause on the monotonous areas of your day and bring some new perspective by changing your actions.

Practice FREE play. Our culture is obsessed with spending money. We do it so well. But I'm going to challenge you to go a full day without spending a dime. You have to actually find joy in moments that are free: picking flowers, planning a light summer picnic in the grass while listening to a free concert in the park, having a viewing night of your favorite show's season finale with friends. Also, consider where you can give back to your community.

Move your body! I can't stress this enough! To own your glow, you need to love your body. Part of loving your body means to move it regularly to keep it healthy. Your workouts are an opportunity for playfulness and self-expression. Swaying your hips in a salsa dance class, bouncing on a rebounder, jumping rope, practicing yoga, grooving through a spin class, scaling a rock-climbing wall, affirming your way through intenSati class, putting on that tennis skirt and hitting the courts, or even light stretching—whatever it is that excites you is what you should be doing.

Be creative! Take an art class. Paint an accent wall in your bedroom. Bake cookies. Start knitting. Get some picture frames and canvases and make collages. Is there something creative you've been wanting to do but have never made time for? Do that!

STIRRING YOUR CREATIVE SAUCE

Now that we know that recreation is a direct pathway to better attunement of our GPS, it's time to use those "aha moments" that result to actively engage with our intuitions and aspirations, opening ourselves up to and better engaging with our GPS to discover what we need to call into our lives. Here are a few suggestions for exercises that will help us stay open and achieve that.

Don't just think it, ink it! Writing down our goals and desires has a peculiar way of activating them in the world. One of the requirements of this book is that you keep a journal so you can write down all your goals, what you desire, and what you are feeling. It gives the Universe a clear indication that you are ready to take your thoughts to the next level and spin them into action.

Love letters. These are letters to that which you wish to create, to help cultivate the creative juices and stir up the powerful force of glow power within you. Write to that dream within, that idea that wants to come forth. Invite it. This will help you to clearly see what you want and help to summon it forth from within. Your desire could take the form of a relationship with a romantic partner, a baby, a business, or a hobby. Write to your desires.

Use your non-dominant hand. Since our hands are connected to our brains, we can stimulate our brains by stimulating our hands—seems simple enough, right? This process utilizes brain plasticity, our brain's ability to change at any age. Brain mapping shows that creativity is housed in the right hemisphere of our brains, so we can stimulate this right brain through working with our left hand. Thankfully, this also works for lefties like me, as studies show that one hemisphere is active when we use our dominant hand, but both hemispheres are activated when we use our non-dominant hand. Write all the ideas that you can think of that encourage your self-expression and doodle.

Color outside the lines. I remember the effort that it took me to stay within the lines while coloring as a young child. This is really a metaphor for life. The restrictions of lines, of imposed structure, can limit our ability to burst beyond the barriers to our creativity. Find a coloring book for kids or adults, grab your Crayola crayons, and allow yourself to get messy.

Mood-Muse Boards

So, you've heard of vision boards. Everyone makes them around the holidays to envision what they want to manifest for the new year. Here is a similar concept stemming from the world of design. A mood board is a visual implement that helps to tell a story, generating emotion and feeling and setting the tone for a designer's collection. The *muse* element is all about inspiration. This is less about putting your dream car, your coveted vacation, or the ideal wedding gown on the board and more about placement of words, colors, and objects that create the mood and tone of your desired life. What do you want your life to *feel* like? What is the mood? This all goes back to the beginning when I asked you to close your eyes. It's your visioning in action. Don't be concerned if it takes you longer than a day to work on this. The idea is that we are stirring the pot of your creativity.

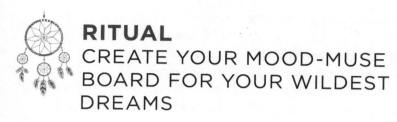

RITUAL
CREATE YOUR MOOD-MUSE BOARD FOR YOUR WILDEST DREAMS

What you will need:

Poster board or stretched canvas, 18" x 24"
Glue stick
Scissors
Markers
Magazines, photographs, found objects

Cut or rip out images that represent your dreams. If one of your dreams is marriage, for instance, rather than focusing on the exact dress, perhaps find an image of a happy couple or two hands clasped or the silhouette of two people standing on the beach. Cut out words and phrases that also resonate. Let your intuition be your guide. There is no wrong or right way to do this; it's pure expression. As you begin to arrange the scraps of paper, step away, then come back and look at it again before you glue everything down. How does it make you feel? Do the imagery and words reflect your inner muse, your wildest dreams? Add or subtract where necessary. When you are ready, glue everything into place. Add any personal design or doodles. Look at your collage often. It's a visual representation of your dreams and gives your GPS images and words to work with. Expect ideas and guidance to result.

Cutting Out the Noise

I recently visited my mom, a huge television buff. I would often find her asleep with the TV on, and I would shut it off every time I entered the room. One particular day, she fell asleep in front of the television again, and when I walked into the room, I heard a report of a young man who had suffered a brutal beating resulting in his death. This information was entering my mother's subconscious mind while she was sleeping. That is frightening. We are not even aware of the mental pollution we welcome into our subconscious mind because we have automatic patterns keeping us from awareness.

Creating space in your life for inspiration in order to better utilize the gift that is our GPS is critical for owning your glow. One impediment to that process is the constant digital chatter that fills our minds. Cutting out the noise and not allowing the technological onslaught we live with daily to interfere with the signal is key. When we are tethered by technology and screen time, it interferes with our GPS. Here are a few ways we can tune out the noise so we can tune within.

TV time out

Put your remote control away. Cut the clutter of programming and commercials out of your life for a few weeks, and during the time you would ordinarily watch television, explore creative projects, cook, organize your space, dive into a spiritual practice, bump up your self-care practice, or spend time in the outdoors. Soul-scribe about the experience of cutting TV out of your life. You may find this becomes your new regular habit.

Try phone-fasting

Turning off the tube isn't enough. Tune all the digital chatter out of your life for one day per week. I know that doing this may send you into a panic attack, and if so, try half a day. Phone-fasting includes not using iPads, computers, video games, and other electronics. Take that time to turn inward; be with yourself or with family. Go for a run, play Frisbee in the park, cuddle with your sweetie and exchange foot massages, cook a meal for someone, write a letter, spend time doing what you love with whomever you love, and take time to appreciate the precious moment that is the present. I promise, you will love being unreachable once you get used to it!

Practice Deep Breathing

Breathing is autonomic and voluntary. You can choose to engage with the breath or not. You can create the state of consciousness you want to achieve through breath. If you're wound up and want to relax, you can breathe your way to relaxation. On the inhale, the nervous system becomes active and stimulated and on the exhale the nervous system becomes calm and centered. Whether seated, standing or lying down, taking a moment to close your eyes and bring your attention to your breath can help you reclaim the present moment and sever the connection to distractions.

What's around the corner?

Your Glow Power System speaks when you least expect it, when you are relaxed and your mind is pliant. That voice is powerful and is strengthened when we trust it and follow it. When we avoid the truth that speaks through that voice, we create disruption—a separation between our inner light and our ambitions. This, in turn, makes us unhappy, moody, less confident. There are consequences for disrespecting our GPS. If you are allowing yourself the time to play while cutting out the distractions that don't serve you but have trouble actively engaging with the whispers that come through, or if you ask your vision question—a reflective query that can help you zero in on what your dream may be communicating—after remembering your dreams and you don't get an answer, it can mean that you may not be quite ready to make the fierce commitment to your inner truth. Aligning our being with our inner truth and recognizing that we are a creative matrix with a divine force is one of our greatest challenges as women. Addressing your inner truth consciously will open up all other doors to creativity in your life.

It's time to stand up and decide what's next in your life. You can either take life as it comes to you or actively participate in molding it, designing it the way you want, with all the bells and whistles to boot. Starting today, you can make the rest of your life enriching, exciting, productive, and stellar. I'm not looking to provide you with a list of things you *should* do but to have you see the exciting possibilities of what you *could* do. You may have an exciting new idea brewing within you or an adventure that's waiting to unfold. What do you really want to do? What do you desire to have? Who do you know you want to be? Where are you itching to go? How do you want to glow in the world?

Be bold and close your eyes. See yourself with all that you desire, standing in your *glow-ry,* and claim it as yours. We have spent this time of self-discovery preparing to craft our mission statements. It's time to move forward in life by calling to us that which will allow us to live our best life—to create that life through the use of our innate glow power. It's not for the Universe to hand over to you, but for you to realize that it's already yours and is waiting just around the corner. Have faith. Turn your "what if" to "what is."

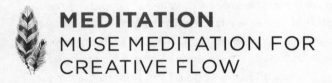

MEDITATION
MUSE MEDITATION FOR CREATIVE FLOW

According to Greek mythos, the Muses traditionally came in the form of nine women. They represented many of the arts and sciences, from poetry to dance to comedy. The Muses gathered and collectively created the concept of the *muse*um and *mus*ic. In this exercise, we honor your muses by writing down and visually depicting your inspiration to keep the channels open. Do this in a place where you find yourself most inspired. For me, it's the ocean. When I am near the beach and in sunshine, I feel my most powerful and inspired. I also find inspiration when in flight and do a lot of my creative visioning in my aisle seat at 37,000 feet. Whenever I find myself stuck, whether it's with writing or developing a program or client service offering, I tune inward for the guidance.

Sit in a quiet place. Light a candle or place a flower or piece of clear quartz in front of you. Turn on music that charges your soul and makes you feel good. Find a comfortable seat. Close your eyes and take 10 long, deep, full belly breaths. Invite your muse in with a request, prayer, or intention. See what images come up during your seated practice. When you open your eyes, write a brief note asking for guidance, insight, and advice for your creative expression. Switch hands and write with your non-dominant hand. Write down or draw what you hear, feel, or intuit. Don't question yourself; it will take you out of the moment. Trust that the muse within, who is governed by your GPS, will emerge with guidance for you.

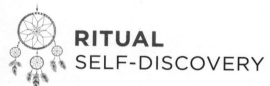

RITUAL
SELF-DISCOVERY

Find a comfortable place to sit. Close your eyes.

Think of all the things you love to do. Visit some old memories for fun. Find your way to the attic of lost dreams, where hope, laughs, quirks, and strengths all exist. Pull out the dust cloth and wipe clean the qualities that have been hidden for so long, captive, because you've been afraid to really be yourself. Journal your answers to these questions truthfully:

What is your unique gift to give?

What do you really love to do that brings you joy?

When you were a child, what did you love to do?

When do you feel divinely inspired?

What do you want to create?

Where do you want to go?

With whom do you want to share?

What would you do if you just couldn't fail?

We wouldn't have an idea swirling in our orbit if it weren't meant to be manifest. Allow yourself the space to expand the idea. Self-expression is allowing the spirit to move through us; it's doing the work we were called to do. Everyone has been made for some particular work, and that work is like medicine that heals.

WITHIN EVERYTHING SACRED THAT EXISTS, I CALL TO CREATIVITY AND ABUNDANCE AND BOW TO IT.

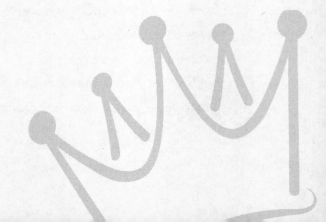

excavation

*"When I let go of what I am, I become what I might be.
When I let go of what I have, I receive what I need."*

~ TAO TE CHING,
ANCIENT CHINESE PHILOSOPHICAL TEXT

I used to live in a beautiful apartment in Harlem. It was located on the neighborhood's most historic block—tree-lined, gorgeous, and world famous for its colorful history and the notable people who'd lived there, such as preacher/congressman Adam Clayton Powell Jr., renowned activist and surgeon Dr. Louis T. Wright, and Bill "Bojangles" Robinson. Even Bob Dylan had owned the building next door to ours many moons ago. I moved in when my son was just five months old and chose to stay there after his father and I split up. But I remember, at the ten-year mark, having a conversation with myself about moving. In truth, I'd been playing with the idea of a new place for a while. I wanted new energy, something with outdoor space. The timing felt good, but I wasn't motivated to do the work of looking for a new apartment.

You see, in theory, I already lived in the perfect place. It was 2,000 square feet with three bedrooms, three fireplaces, two bathrooms, a walk-in pantry, a washer and dryer, a full living room, and a dining room. It was the type of place you don't move from, that you keep in the family. Half of my neighbors had lived most of their lives in that building, one of them for 65 years. And yet, something was telling me to go.

But I rolled into my 11th year living in this beautiful space, not having searched for a new one. And so it was, two days before Thanksgiving, that my son and I left our home together and headed downtown on our routine commute, first him to school, then me to my office. A mere hour later, I got a phone call. Our apartment building was on fire. I was flooded with emotion but calmly called neighbors to be sure everyone was safe and exiting the building. Thankfully, everyone escaped; the damage, however, was devastating.

When I arrived back, it looked like a war zone. The firemen had needed to bust through every door and destroy windows to isolate the fire. No one was allowed to stay there. I was escorted in by the chief of the department of buildings just so I could collect some things to take with me. I had to wear a mask to enter the unlit building. There was no electricity or gas. Glass shards were everywhere, and murky, muddy water mixed with sand covered the floors as I made my way up to the fourth. A dank blanket of smoke filled the apartment, and all my clothes smelled like I had been sitting around a campfire for days on end. I gathered what I needed and packed our lives into suitcases and a duffel bag, having no idea where I would be going.

My son and I lived out of those suitcases in a sublet through the winter as our landlords dragged their feet on repairs. But I saw clearly that beneath this new challenge I was facing was an opportunity. I needed to see it as a spiritual growth spurt. I'm a Taurus and stubborn by nature, so much so that the Universe thrusts me into situations that spark change because I would probably not seek the change on my own. The devastation we faced was clearing the space for something new, for abundance, and because I couldn't take the leap on my own to move, God had removed me from my circumstances and was opening the door for new energy, opportunity and the chance for a new home.

I found a new place at just the right time—spring, with its ushering in of new beginnings. It felt good to clear out 11 years of my life. What was truly cluttering my apartment, and therefore my life, were the remnants of my past relationship. I needed to move on. I was in a new relationship with a loving partner who showed me his deep capacity for love as he supported me every step of the way through this shift. I needed a push in letting go so that I could make space for the life that awaited me. The physical manifestations and memories were everywhere, and it seemed I would never sort it all out.

With the help of Marie Kondo's international bestselling book *The Life-Changing Magic of Tidying Up: The Japanese Art of Decluttering and Organizing*, I breezed through the sorting, saving, organizing, and giving away of many of my belongings. I got new furnishings and started fresh. I went from living in a prewar walk-up to a newly constructed building with an elevator. And although sometimes I miss the stairs, I don't miss the commute. I can walk my son to school three blocks away, walk to my office, and spend quiet mornings on the rooftop or meditate on New York City's High Line among the plants. The Universe really had this worked out!

Sometimes God will move a perceived obstacle that you can't move on from on your own—a job, a relationship, a beautiful home. And sometimes we need to do the work of identifying those obstacles ourselves—be they harmful ideas, behaviors, or even people—and then let them go. Just think: when you travel, you pack a bag to carry. But what if you never unpacked it and just kept accumulating things along the way? Eventually, you would run out of space. Now, imagine that these physical bags contain aspects of your life, your *personal* baggage. Do you want to carry every little thing that's happened to you—stuff all the heartbreak, hardship, the good times, the upsets, and the drama—into compartments? Do you really want to take all that with you everywhere you go? We are walking manifestations of our karma. Every experience and decision we have made up to this point has shaped who we are. However, that does not mean we have to physically carry the baggage of past experiences with us.

When we dwell in our trauma, when we engage in dysfunctional relationships or addictive patterns, we dial into our fear system big-time, shutting down our GPS. That GPS was put there to guide us to our highest potential, to help us see the way. It's easy to keep living a life without challenging yourself, but we all have spiritual growth spurts that need to be addressed, and altering the relationships and behaviors in your life will help you see how critical personal-growth work really is. By lugging our baggage around, we stifle our glow power and dim our own light. We limit our ability to call into our orbit that specific thing we decided to aim for. We cut ourselves off from our personal mission.

We want to stay on mission, and to stay the course, we must excavate. You want to maneuver through life smoothly, amplify that GPS, allow for personal growth, and take only what you can carry by yourself—just enough to fit in the overhead compartment. So, as you examine your baggage, what do you need to unpack and leave behind?

Some things were right for us at a particular time but are no longer serving our higher purpose and become a hindrance to our growth. And some things that we allow to anchor in our lives were toxic from the beginning—be they feelings of fear, self-doubt, grudges and resentment, toxic relationships, harmful behaviors and influences, or the baggage, both emotional and physical, of past trauma. In this chapter we'll explore what is weighing us down, and we'll work to let it go.

PERSONAL GROWTH IS NOT ABOUT HOW MUCH YOU ACCUMULATE BUT HOW MUCH YOU RELEASE.

It's time to unpack the bags, honey. So, what's eating you? What in your life is pulling you under? Are you unhappy with your sur-roundings? Any dissatisfaction you are experiencing, anything that is eating away at you, is a product of your current patterning. It's been placed in your life for a purpose, and you chose it—maybe not consciously, but you made a choice nonetheless. How can you unhook yourself from this environment?

Are there people who don't belong in your life, though you wish things were different? When we are free from the "BS" we have allowed to enter our lives, we have the freedom to create. Who needs to be removed from your inner circle?

Let's be clear—some of the things you need to let go of are going to draw up a lot of emotion because they have taproots laid deep down within us. But what you need for healing is already present within you—you were born with it—and we are clearing the obstacles so you can hear it full blast. Slow down, be still, and start listening.

In the recesses of darkness lie our shadow aspects, things we want to disassociate from or may even be unconscious of, things we don't want others to see or know about ourselves. The shadow reflects some of the negative aspects of ourselves and our behaviors. But in order to really shine in the world, it's critical to dig deep and excavate your dark side. I don't mean disown it. Rather, open it up, see what's inside, and own it. And acknowledge that our shadow aspects can hold us back. We want to bring it to light and begin to release the behaviors that perpetuate these patterns of playing small, negative self-dialogue, putting our priorities on the back burner, and stewing in circumstances that no longer work in our favor. What truths are you ready to see about yourself now?

Digging in the Darkness

Taking this journey requires us to be deeply engaged in inquiry that reveals our true nature and the blocks we have to fulfilling our potential. And often, we don't want to ask the juicy questions because we fear we'll find something that we don't want to know or don't have the capacity to fix. But when we truly desire and are ready to grow ourselves beyond who we are, then asking questions becomes a huge catalyst in our quest for transformation. Empowering questions will give you the ability to make the best choices, thus facilitating the change you seek in your life. I encourage you to start asking yourself probing and productive questions to unlock hidden tendencies and obstacles and identify parts of yourself that need a little more glow.

When you construct your questions, use "the Core Four": *who, what, when,* and *how.*

Who am I holding on to by attracting people who don't serve my highest good?

What do I gain by remaining stuck in the same situation or circumstances?

When do I feel my best, and what is keeping me from following that feeling?

How have I constructed my life to follow other people's rules?

Avoid using *why*, because it automatically puts us on the defensive and sets us up for a punitive or shaming experience of inquiry rather than one that's educational, informative, and in depth. Notice the difference in energy between the following two questions:

Why don't people respect me at work?

How can I better assert myself so I feel respected at work?

Airing Out Your Fears

As you continue this line of self-exploration, asking questions, and checking in with your body, you may observe patterns of self-destructiveness, depression, danger, or addiction. Have you met your inner saboteur? What are the ways you sabotage yourself?

Rather than chastising yourself for what you discover, start to think about those behaviors from a perspective of discovery. How can you use this information in an investigative way? *What are you gaining by behaving in a certain way?* Most often, our sabotaging behaviors are really a protective mechanism against what we fear. Whatever the behavior, almost always the answer is that you are harboring self-doubt and feeling afraid. We must begin to face the attachments we have to entertaining harmful behavior. We must examine how we create sabotaging imprints by engaging in chaotic situations and holding space for addictive environments.

We are attached to the idea that our feelings and anxiety are a reflection of situations we are already in, but the truth is quite the opposite. Our fear is in fact attracting the very situations and people that justify our fear-based beliefs. Fear is a resistance to the ebb and flow of life, and our lives need to be fluid. How many times have you allowed the fear of not getting what you want in life, the fear of being hurt, rejected, disappointed, or abandoned, dictate your actions and stop you from taking risks? Now it is time to fully acknowledge the fears that have been paralyzing you and robbing you of joy, opportunity, growth, and love. Growth is uncomfortable because it requires us to shake ourselves from the clutching structure of our lives. We must deconstruct and dethrone our fear, seize our rightful crowns as queens, consecrate our visions, and take dominion over our own lives.

Your Capacity to Receive

Many of our behavioral patterns suggest that we don't believe that we should receive what's coming our way. Over the years I have had to adjust my relationship with having and holding what I have asked for. Some of us believe we can't really have what we want, although we recite mantras and prayers stating otherwise. Some of us believe we are destined to be alone, or we will never have financial security. Even if you are underresourced right now, you are in control of your thoughts and can jump-start a new thought pattern. We design our lives around these narratives of doubt and sabotage ourselves consciously and unconsciously because we believe there is a fixed amount of happiness or success we can actually achieve. Let's check in with your capacity to receive. Soul scribe on the following questions:

In what ways do I need to expand my capacity to receive?

Where do I need to take up more space in my life?

What is my relationship to having? Do I feel deserving?

What are the harmful patterns I fall back on when I feel uncomfortable receiving?

Where can I challenge my comfort and grow into a healthier relationship with having more?

Having cleared the baggage, what risks will I take?

Boundless Beliefs Soul Scribe

If you stay rooted in your purpose and focused on the unique contributions only you can make to the world, you will find that the benevolent Universe will support your action. There are many ways you can effect change as well as inspire it: being a leader in your home or community, raising incredible children, launching a business or creating a product that solves a problem in the world, volunteering to help others. The only impediments to your success are the beliefs you hold and the perceptions you carry about yourself and what's possible. I refer to limiting beliefs as binding beliefs because they hold us back and keep us from expanding and growing. In this exercise, we're going to take the "Core Four" a step further and journal for a few paragraphs or pages and turn our limiting or binding beliefs into boundless ones. We are going to transform our inner dialogue.

Soul-scribe freely on your limitations. You can complain, reveal your fears, or write about anything else you might feel the urge to do to help free yourself.

You can write simple sentences, but I encourage you to expand upon them if you have more to say. You can do this for however many fears or binding beliefs surface for you. For example:

I fear that I am incapable of running a successful company as an entrepreneur.

Because I did not grow up with models of success and there is so much pressure on me to change the legacy and be the successful one in the family, I don't want to let everyone down.

I feel powerless when I let this feeling take over.

I know that I have to work on my self-sabotaging tendencies and embrace my power.

If you need help getting started, use these prompts:

I fear _____

Because _____

I feel _____

I know _____

Now that you have your soul scribe complete, I want you to take some time now to write down a list of just the binding beliefs on one side of the page, and for each, come up with the opposing thought—the positive, affirmative statement that transforms your binding belief to a boundless one. Once you have this list, you can create beautiful note cards or leave sticky notes with these affirmations around for yourself as constant reminders.

For example:

I fear that I am incapable of running a successful company as an entrepreneur.

becomes

I believe that I am capable of running a successful company as an entrepreneur and know that owning my abilities and embracing my power will help me achieve my goals.

Imagine what would happen if you spent some time really deconstructing your binding beliefs in all areas of your life and reframed your inner dialogue. You would be unstoppable!

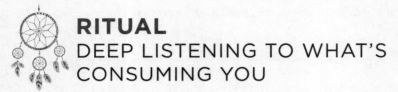

RITUAL
DEEP LISTENING TO WHAT'S CONSUMING YOU

For some, it might help to listen to the body to engage and observe what comes to the surface. Our emotions are very peculiar and are often lodged away within our living tissues, becoming part of us. We store our psychic pain physically in our bodies. For each emotion, there is a space within our bodies that tethers it. Here is a technique that I use to check in when I need grounding. It's a ritual that requires you to be still and vulnerable with yourself. It's not about succumbing to the compulsion to control what is happening around you and within you, and it's not about trying to fix anything—you aren't broken. This is an opportunity to simply listen, acknowledge, and accept where you are right now.

Start by finding a comfortable surface where you can set the tone for the space. Place a drop of your favorite essential-oil blend or flower essence on your wrists and temples or use a diffuser so the scent fills the room. Lie down flat on your back. I usually use my bed or a yoga mat and place a small towel underneath my sacrum (the small, or lower part, of the back). You want to assume full savasana *pose, with your legs fully extended and your arms alongside your body with palms face-up. Close your eyes and deepen your breath. Scan your body. Feel where there might be any tension.*

Ask yourself:

Where in my body am I sensing tension?

Am I feeling anger?

When I focus on fear, where does it show up in my body?

While you lie there, I want you to imagine yourself fully supported in this process. All you have to do is close your eyes, breathe, and focus on what you feel when you speak to your body. This is a way to connect sensation with emotion and allow your body to speak back. There may be some questions you want to ask yourself more specifically. When we shed light on our fears, they lose power over us and we can choose to transform them and see them in a new light. We can let them go.

What You're Consuming

We are shifting from what's consuming us, the opinions and ideals and pain inflicted by others, to what we are consuming of negative influence, most notably through the media, both traditional and social.

There are lots of toxic messages pervasive in the media; they add stress to our lives and take us out of the moment. When our minds are running rampant with negative thoughts related to media messages, we are not mentally or emotionally available for blessings or breakthroughs. The stress keeps us in a belief system that thrives on scarcity. We start to believe the messages of "I am not enough. I don't have enough," and that can send us spiraling in some cases. Think about the messages you are ingesting through traditional media—print, television, the radio, books, or movies. How do you feel after reading a high fashion or beauty magazine? Do you start to criticize your thighs or imagine your hair a different texture and length?

There are pervasive negative body images and harmful messaging about sexuality and race that we are confronted with at every turn. Change up your traditional media by simply supporting magazines, books, blogs, and podcasts that reflect your lifestyle goals. Listen to inspirational podcasts while you're on-the-go to help motivate you.

Reality television can seed ideas about how to function in relationships and promote catty behavior and petty drama among women. The news gives us traumatic messaging about current events and fuels the fear that no one and no place is safe. We can't lead our lives with our heads stuck in the sand, but we don't have to subject ourselves to toxic messaging, either. Instead of vegetating in the latest reality star's drama, why not prioritize your programming?

Use a streaming service and select from a wider range of content. If your goal is to start an interior-design business, find some inspirational YouTube channels focused on design and follow them. Streamline the news you get on your mobile device so you control what you see and when.

And what about your Twitter and Facebook feeds? What messages are you getting via Instagram? Are you following mean-girl accounts, or do you like empowerment-focused pages? Social media can be a powerful tool but a cruel master. The beauty of it is that you can create the world in which you want to play. You can connect selectively with people online, form new virtual communities, and control what you see to a certain extent. You can filter what you want to share and see so that you only see accounts that uplift you. The blocking feature on your social channels is powerful—do not be shy to use it when you are dealing with internet trolls. When in doubt, block. It will prevent a barrage of pettiness from seeping into your life. Do a virtual edit to check in twice a year with your social-media pages and add accounts that you find very motivating and uplifting. Delete pages that cultivate insecurity, judgment, and self-doubt dialogue in you.

Couldn'ts, Won'ts, Shouldn'ts, and Don'ts

Do you have a tiny voice in your head that directs you from a negative standpoint? "You shouldn't do that. Don't eat this. You can't. That won't work." So many of us are plagued by the cacophony of discouraging words speaking to us through the lens of self-doubt. Why do we always tell ourselves *no* and start managing our expectations for excellence before we set foot on the journey? In some part of ourselves, we feel inadequate. This experience is normal for most women in modern society, but it is certainly not acceptable. Stop *shoulding* yourself. Start *being* yourself. When you *should* yourself, it's to conform to someone else's ideal, an archetype of who they expect you to be, how they expect you to act. You are putting constraints on yourself, constricting growth, impeding learning, and nourishing planted seeds of doubt, allowing them to take root.

Beloved, when you are being yourself, you break the mold. You construct the archetypes and shape-shift through them, you create space for personal growth, you become a scholar of the self, and you find healing, sowing the seeds of self-love. When you begin to love yourself instead of doubt yourself, everything shifts around you, from the way people perceive you and interact with you to the circumstances and situations you attract. The first person you must fall in love with is you. That is your holiest relationship. That is where the forgiveness starts: with you and from within.

Freedom to Forgive

Why is it important to forgive? When hanging on to past transgressions, we cloud our GPS. To forgive is to make a conscious choice to free yourself from the fear, tension, and pain cycle associated with the dramas and traumas of life. Forgiveness offers you the gift of levity—feeling lighter and having emotional and spiritual mobility. You are not tethered by pains that haunt you. Forgiveness constantly invites us to be healed and, like anything else that is meaningful and impactful in our lives, it can take time. Forgiveness also offers us wisdom that we can apply to future situations. We can look back and extract nuggets of knowledge and be grateful we were able to learn and grow so much.

On a physiological level, there are places in the body where our anger, trauma, and resentment reside. These emotions create blockages that deny us full access to our storehouse of creative energy—our glow power. I know you have gone through some tough things in your life. You have suffered, and I am sure there are some people in your life whom you need to forgive. There may be some people who you wish would forgive you. A weepy, tear-filled apology may not be accepted but needs to be expressed nonetheless. Forgiveness does not mean you condone a certain action or celebrate bad behavior. Instead, you are reclaiming your well-being, standing up, and saying, *"I will no longer carry this heavy load. My heart is too big to be weighed down by woes. I choose to let this go."*

As we become more skillful at practicing forgiveness, the heavy load we have been carrying becomes lighter, and eventually we can toss it to the wind.

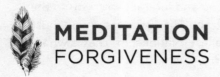

MEDITATION
FORGIVENESS

To ease yourself into a practice of forgiveness, I invite you to try this meditation. Settle into a quiet space. You may want to light a candle or burn incense to set the mood.

Find a comfortable seated position, and if you are flexible, lie back onto pillows so that your chest is open. Gently close your eyes and breathe. Breathe gently into your heart space, notice where you feel any tension or restriction. Are you able to breathe deeply? Allow yourself to feel the narrowing walls of the fortress created by the weight of the emotions you have carried for so long. As you breathe, become aware of any constriction around your heart. Forgiveness allows us to breathe with ease. Inhale and begin asking yourself for forgiveness and extend forgiveness from your own heart to others who have caused you pain.

Turn your attention to your own precious body and life. Let yourself begin to visualize the ways you have hurt or have been unkind to yourself. Allow any sensations of pain or sorrow you have been carrying with you come to the surface, and release yourself of these burdens. Extend forgiveness to yourself for each of them.

Forgiveness Mantra to release myself from myself: I have wronged myself, intentionally and unknowingly, through abuse or abandonment, through words or harsh actions.

I forgive myself. I'm ready to let this go.

Take a moment to visualize the ways you may have hurt others. Acknowledge the pain you have caused out of your own fear. Tap into your own genuine sorrow. Know that you can release this burden and ask for forgiveness. Picture each memory that still burdens your heart. Are you ready to let it go and move forward?

Forgiveness Mantra to release myself from those I have hurt: *I have wronged people in my life, intentionally and unknowingly, through abuse or abandonment, through words or harsh actions.*

I ask for your forgiveness.

Allow yourself to visualize the ways others have wronged you, causing pain or confusion. Feel the sorrow you have carried from past and know that now you can release this burden of pain by extending forgiveness when your heart is ready.

Forgiveness Mantra to release those who have hurt me: *I have been wronged by people in my life, intentionally and unknowingly, through abuse or abandonment, through words or harsh actions.*

I have carried this pain far too long. I wish to move on. I offer my forgiveness. To those who have caused me harm, I offer my forgiveness. I forgive you.

Let yourself gently repeat these three mantras of forgiveness while in deep visualization until you start to feel a release in your heart. You may find you're not quite ready to let go and move on; be gentle with yourself. Forgiveness is not something I can force upon you. I can only encourage you to continue the practice of softening to your vulnerability and let the words and visualizations work to open your heart.

Mantras of Resentment

When we speak negatively about anything, we affirm that negative vibration as a truth. Be mindful of your statements about yourself and others: "I'm so stupid," "I hate her," "He makes me sick," "I'm a mess." These statements fly out of our mouths without much thought. And these negativities can build upon one another to form our own personal mantras of resentment.

I once dated a man I thought I would marry. We were so in love and so excited about what lay ahead that we were already living in the promise of a future together. The courtship was intense, but as soon as our souls decided the time was right, his ego went rogue. He started exhibiting odd behaviors. He was afraid. He felt he needed to escape, and fast. And so he did.

I was left confused and aching, with my heart pried open, pulsing and wounded. A blanket of sadness overcame me. I didn't know how to process the loss of true love. I couldn't seem to let go of the fact that "He hurt me. He didn't protect my emotions." I had never loved someone so deeply, and I resented him for the pain he had caused me. I ignored him when he came crawling back to be near me. I put up walls and shunned him for not stepping up in the way I thought he should. I was afraid to be vulnerable, to be hurt again, so I wore my resentment as a suit of armor.

Sometime later, I met a girlfriend for lunch. We hadn't seen each other in a while; she wanted the full update on my life, work, and love. But I decided in that moment, before launching into my well-worn story of heartbreak, that I was done speaking about it. Done speaking about the loss. Done making that person out to be a bad guy. I was done firing up the neuropathways of pain and reliving the experience on a cellular level each and every time I spoke about it. I was done being upset and carrying that feeling in my heart. I wanted to dial back up my radiance and just let it go. I wanted to open myself up to a new story. He had written me tons of letters, which I had tossed as they arrived, but one day, I wrote him back. I wrote a letter full of love for myself. I spoke my truth, I shared my feelings, I affirmed what I deserve, and I released it. I did not expect him to respond, nor did I *want* a response. I had decided to do it for my healing alone and to let myself off the hook by practicing forgiveness.

From that moment onward, I felt a rush of warmth come over me, a peace in my being. I was no longer carrying the baggage or uttering mantras of resentment toward him or myself. I could breathe with ease and felt lighthearted again. I even became a major magnet for men because the energy around me was light, not weighed down by baggage or dismissive vibes. I didn't need to dwell on "the one that got away." That story line only made him out to be a bad guy and made me a victim. It kept me living in the past. With forgiveness, I could now make space for a new partner who would come into my life to enhance it, to help me on my quest to continue to grow and own my glow.

Ditch Your Stinking Thinking

In your journal, write down how many times you utter statements that fall into the resentment category. Keep the log for at least a full day. Notice how many times you make unvoiced comments to yourself about yourself and others. Explore these resentments beneath the surface. Whom are you upset with? More important, what negative patterns are you perpetuating because this person has not *earned* your forgiveness? What small steps can you take toward letting go?

Weeding Your Garden

Maxwell, a Grammy Award–winning recording artist and dear friend, taught me a very special lesson once about fierce boundaries and letting go of toxic relationships. One day, long after I'd met him, he called to personally give me his new phone number. When I asked why he was going through such an effort to change a number that he'd had for ages, he said, "I'm just weeding out the wackness, clearing out my social garden, so to speak, so all that's left are flowers." I loved this metaphor, since I liken everything in life to flowers and gardens. Clearing out the weeds of unhealthy relationships is an important step in preparing ourselves for the next phase of our personal development and creating protective space around what we are dreaming about most.

If you look at your life like a garden and see every living thing in that garden as either supporting the cultivation of your best self or strangling all the goodness that is thriving in your life, then you will very quickly identify what belongs and what does not. Imagine that your personal relationships make up the elements of the garden. Some plants work well together and support each other's growth. Other plants, like weeds, cut through the goodness and create trouble for the garden. In a garden, when the oxygen does not flow, the surrounding plants suffer and often die. You might have relationships that function more like weeds and cause constriction where there should be flow. We've all had moments when we've felt stifled. Think of a time in your life when you've felt that way; maybe there are a few. When you aren't allowing the oxygen to flow freely, it's an indication that you aren't breathing properly and likely experiencing stress.

Some of us have friends in our lives who are simply unsupportive. You know, the ones who bash your goals with criticism, who somehow don't want to see you win—someone who makes you doubt you're doing the right thing or making the right decision. Sure, these "friends" commiserate with you on your worst days, but they are envious when you are having your best days. You've invested so much in your friendships that you're sensitive about letting go. Are you looking to change the energy around you but nervous about losing friends? That's a fear that so many women carry: "What if I alienate the people I care about?"

Sometimes for the sake of our personal growth, we have to cut ties to people so we can move to the next phase of our development. It's said, "You are the company you keep."

Why not examine all the relationships you are a part of and then nourish the ones that are sustaining and weed out (or at least send less oxygen to) the ones that are less fulfilling? You have to be able to distinguish who your true friends are. You need to know that you are safe. Where are the weeds entwined in your friendships? Who in your circle is planting seeds of doubt? If you're someone who has been prone to cattiness and competition in the past, drawn in by a crowd of mean girls, I encourage you to closely monitor your social groups and activities for that kind of energy.

So, how do you know if someone belongs in your trusted-sister circle? Ask yourself the following questions about that person. The answers should all be a resounding *yes*!

Does spending time with this person lift me up?

Does she make me a better person?

Am I happy in her company?

Am I allowed to be myself in this friendship?

Does she celebrate my successes?

Does she tell me the truth, even if it's uncomfortable?

Does she help me to grow?

Does she own her glow?

If the answers to these questions are *no*, then what can you do to remedy the situation? You've identified the relationship as unhealthy or unsustainable. We can focus on less contact with the people in our lives who don't make a positive impact. You may choose to have a conversation with each person or simply change your own actions. Become more involved in your personal journey and invest your time and energy in relationships that support your growth and help you move forward on your path. You become whomever you surround yourself with.

Combatting the Good-Girl Conditioning

Tuck your shirt in, tie your shoes, cross your legs, smile big—but not too big—nod your head, fold your hands, shhh . . . be quiet. Be a good girl. The dichotomy of good and bad in our culture is perverse when it comes to traditional gender roles and idealized feminine behavior. The exalted good girl is cheery, simpleminded, obedient, approval-seeking, childlike yet upright, and, in recent years, well educated. The bad girl is the polar opposite—promiscuous, dark, rebellious, sensual, careless or carefree, attention-seeking. No one really wants to be known for those "bad girl" traits, but who really wants to *be* the "good girl"? Many of us have had to play the role of the "goody-goody" our whole lives. As a child seeking the approval of your parents, it made sense to want to be good. As a freethinking, grown woman who wants to live her own life, however, you don't need to please anyone but yourself. It's time to let go of the "good girl" complex.

Have you ever thought about what your life would look like if you were concerned only with *you* feeling good about your decisions? Let's face it, some of your decisions are going to piss other people off. Are you okay with that? Because you need to be focused on pleasing yourself first, no longer bound by the opinions of others, no longer living your life at the expense of your emotional and spiritual freedom. Being a fully realized woman is not about making grown-up decisions that let everyone else off the hook. When you let go of being that good girl, you can succeed beyond measure, because you will no longer be tied down to what you previously thought was possible through the lens of what others thought was possible for you.

The little girl within wants to win validation, but for us to step into roles of leadership in our work and in our lives, we have to get comfortable with the idea that not everyone is going to like us. That's just the truth. Remember, instead, that you have potency. Rise in that. To lead with grace and not defer to someone else's authority is to own your glow. It's not about being a good girl. Disobedience breeds discovery—self-discovery.

Disobedience is about having audacity. When you break the mold and change the course others have set out for you, a whole new world awaits. Not only do you discover the depths of your power, you also learn how to use it in your favor. If you always follow the rules and do as you're told, you may never reach your highest potential because you're not pushed to your edge. Sometimes achieving excellence requires you to step out on faith and go against the grain.

Take a look at women, historical and contemporary, whom we cherish and are fascinated by: Harriet Tubman, Joan of Arc, Rosa Parks, Sojourner Truth, Gloria Steinem, Oprah Winfrey. Their stories are about rising up, standing up, speaking up, shaking things up, resilience. Saying no. Being badass. Being conduits for change. We come from a legacy of strong women.

There are names of women whose stories we know well, and some are tucked away in history books like Mary Ann Shadd Cary, the second black female attorney in the USA who organized the Colored Women's Progressive Franchise Association in 1880. Naomi Anderson, a suffragist whose controversial speech at the first Women's Rights Convention in Chicago in 1869 set the crowd ablaze. Or Ida B. Wells, who founded the Chicago-based Alpha Suffrage Club. Or Angelina Grimké, an abolitionist and women's rights activist who dedicated her life to publishing incisive arguments to end slavery and to advance women's rights. What about Anna Julia Cooper, who once said, "The old, subjective, stagnant, indolent, and wretched life for woman has gone. She has as many resources as men, as many activities beckon her on. As large possibilities swell and inspire her heart"? These accomplished women mobilized people and moved mountains, sometimes using civil disobedience to make their point.

Not all of history's women embraced these ideals of equality, and not all women have been interested in change.

> The moment woman begins to feel the promptings of ambition, or the thirst for power, her aegis of defense is gone. All the sacred protections of religion, all the generous promptings of chivalry, all the poetry of romantic gallantry, depend upon woman's retaining her place as dependent and defenseless, and making no claims, and maintaining no right but what are the gifts of honor, rectitude and love.
>
> *- Catherine Beecher Stowe*

Catherine Beecher Stowe was an education advocate and the sister of Harriet Beecher Stowe. The piece above is an excerpt from her response to Angelina Grimké's public plea for women to aid in abolitionist efforts. Beecher believed that women held a quiet but powerful influence within the family and home. She stressed that for a woman to take a public stance on a political issue was "out of her appropriate sphere." In other words, she held fast to the archetype of the good girl. But Grimké and countless others recognized the importance of women as defiant leaders in the public sphere.

What if women had never taken a stand against slavery? What if we'd never fought for our right to vote? What if we'd never stood up for equal rights? What if our ancestors had instead kept meek, with their mouths shut? What would our world look like today? We might have never seen the likes of Angela Davis; First Lady Michelle Obama; Malala Yousafzai; Sheryl Sandberg; Black Lives Matter co-founders Opal Tometi, Alicia Garza, and Patrisse Cullors; esteemed Supreme Court Justice Sonia Sotomayor; feisty congresswoman Maxine Waters; or our first female nominee for U.S. president by one of our two major political parties, Hillary Clinton.

We might never have seen the day when women would come together to march on Washington and around the world in record numbers in solidarity and support of one another to speak out against injustice and in defense of our rights as we did on January 21, 2017. Each of us can use our power like Tamika D. Mallory, Carmen Perez, Linda Sarsour, and Bob Bland did to organize and lead the Women's March on Washington with the collaborative support of thousands of women and male allies. It all started with an intention, a passionate cry, commitment, and action.

Each of us comes from a lineage of strength. We have pedigree and power, but it's usually tucked away and seldom utilized because we are afraid of being "unlikable," afraid of saying something that might offend. We are afraid of speaking truth to power. Own your opinion and your ideas. Speak your truth. Take action. Be you. Be authentic. Getting over wanting everyone to like you will free you to do what you were put on this planet to do in the first place.

Sometimes people don't like you because you're a woman, or you're too tall, or too smart, or too ethnic, too urban, too preppy, too pretty. Sometimes people don't like you because they can't *be* you. You have to be willing to be alone to become a leader. Sometimes you are the *only* one on your mission. Your cosmic imprint is important. When you commit to your mission, even if you feel alone, a fleet of Earth angels will appear to help you get through it. My grandmother says, "If God will lead you to it, God will get you through it."

Examining Your Good-Girl Conditioning

Many of us operate with an inner dialogue that stems from the need to be accepted and liked. On a daily basis, we consciously and unconsciously compete for male attention and affirmation. Acceptance and likability were actually mechanisms for survival when women did not always have the resources, rights, education, safety, economic mobility, and voice to speak up and do for themselves as we do today. If women did not have the approval and support of those who were in a position to provide for them, it could result in stressful and potentially devastating outcomes. In many parts of the world, women are still living like this—with very little in the way of resources and completely dependent upon and beholden to oppressive influences. We've collectively been holding on to this pattern for generations—it's now part of our operating system. But how can we delete it? What feels worse: to bend and morph into the good girl or to face the fear and reverse this conditioning?

Take out your journal and answer the following questions:

- What have I been taught about being nice?

- How have I prioritized others before myself in a detrimental way?

- What have I been criticized about that mirrored my own beliefs about myself?

- Was there an instance in my life where I went against the grain and spoke up for myself and was met with resistance?

- What have I seen happen to other women that has amplified my fear about speaking up?

- How much does what others think about my appearance matter to me?

Notice what patterns emerge in your answers. What attachments do you have to these thought patterns? Don't worry if you're not quite ready to cut the cord. This is an ongoing reflective practice of excavating deep-rooted beliefs and reprogramming ourselves for greatness.

Revisit this page in your journal when you get to the smudging exercise for a clearance-and-release ritual.

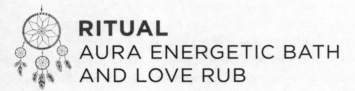

RITUAL
AURA ENERGETIC BATH
AND LOVE RUB

A spiritual cleansing bath is a powerful way to melt away stress, banish stagnant energy or thoughts, and clear your aura. Your aura is an energetic mirror of your physical body. The aura carries an accumulation of thoughts, ideas, beliefs, emotions, and intentions. Throughout the day you accumulate energy from the people and places you have encountered.

Sea salt is used for spiritual cleansing. Salt also has a detoxifying quality that draws out impurities in the energy bodies and the cells. Or, you can substitute Epsom salt for sea salt; it is high in magnesium, easing aches, pains, and the muscles. Consider adding 20 drops of essential oil to the bath if you'd like.

Run a warm bath, adding in a handful of sea salt. As you soak, begin to envision pure, white light; imagine any negative vibrations hovering around the aura being absorbed by this light.

After the salt bath, anoint yourself with a rich body oil or butter. With firm and intentional touch, rub the oil into your skin, self-massaging your entire body. Spend extra time with the areas that don't regularly receive your touch, perhaps your thighs, outer hips, breasts, and belly. Self-massage increases circulation, soothes the nervous system, and affirms the body through loving touch.

Clearing the Physical Space

Now we move from the space of being influenced by the messages we receive to the messages we send ourselves in the form of the refuse lingering in our lives. We hold on to things that often contribute to holding us back. Where might you be storing the physical manifestations and energy of the past in your present life—be they traumatic, harmless but just taking up space, or just no longer fruitful? Clearing the physical space is an important step in excavation.

Sometimes we are holding on to things that would be a blessing in someone else's life. My friend Mara Brock Akil told me once that she used to hate cleaning out her closet and avoided it at all costs. She finally cleared her closet and there was a beautiful purse that was nearly brand new that she knew was no longer meant for her; it was meant for her assistant. So she gifted her assistant the purse and something about that transmission of energy flipped a switch for that young lady.

Whether it's your bedroom, a cluttered closet, an old purse, your desk, or a vintage sofa, the things that take up space in your life have an impact on you.

- **Clear out old relationships.** Remnants of past relationships still perforate the present, and their lingering energy requires that you take some practical action. Are you holding on to nostalgic pieces of days past? Do you still have your ex's old T-shirts stuffed away somewhere? Clean them all out!

- **Clean out your closets.** Move through your bedroom and closets, and let go of remnants of the past. Only keep the clothes or special items that bring you joy. If you find something you haven't worn in nine months, give it away. My fiancé always says, "When in doubt, throw it out." Or you can bless someone else with your old items. Clearing them is essential for you to create more space for what's to come.

- **Downsize your handbag.** Carry a smaller handbag. It trains you to carry only what is essential for your well-being and what you truly need for the day. When you carry only what you need to feel and look radiant, you will begin to mirror that energetically. Some of us have to clear our purses to invite in the abundance we desire in our lives. In some cases, it may mean getting a brand-new purse. As Erykah Badu says in her neosoul classic song "Bag Lady," "I guess nobody ever told you, all you must hold on to is you."

- **Smudge.** In some ancient and native cultures, incense, sage, and resins are burned during rituals both to symbolize prayers, which are believed to be carried to the Creator along the rising smoke, and to bring about visions, amplified by the scent. But this process, known as smudging, is equally if not more well-known for its purification purposes. Smudging is used to purify tools and people, to "wash off" the influences of the outside world before important spiritual ceremonies. It can clear sacred spaces and provide an opening in the soul before summoning spiritual energy. Objects or spaces are likewise washed off with sage-medicine smoke to rid them of unwanted energies. We might smudge a room or ourselves after heavy healing work, when someone is ill, after an argument, or after the disruptive energy of visitors in our homes or offices. Smudging will be a crucial element of the cleansing rituals we explore; consider it spiritual disinfectant.

Herbs for Clearance Rituals

Sweetgrass is considered the sacred hair of Mother Earth; its sweet aroma reminds people of the gentle, clean breeze. Native Americans collect it and braid it into three strands representing love, kindness, and honesty—all qualities of the Earth Mother. This very special herb carries a sweet, vanilla-like scent and is burned to remind us of the feminine essence and that the earth and soil provide and sustain us with everything we need. Sweetgrass is used for smudging and purification of the spirit. When sweetgrass is used in a healing or talking circle, it has a calming effect. It is said to attract positivity and grounding in the divine feminine.

Cedar trees are very old. They hold wisdom and house powerful spirits. Like sage and sweetgrass, cedar is used to purify the home, apartment, or office, often upon first moving in. Cedar also has many restorative medicinal uses; it is a medicine of protection. When mixed with sage for a tea, it helps to cleanse the body of all infections. Cedar baths are also very healing.

Lavender is often mixed into smudge wands. Lavender has wonder powers of protection and cleansing. Traditionally, it has been used in herbal medicine to combat infectious diseases and has soothing effect on the nervous system. Lavender brings a positive energy, opens the heart chakra, and calms the busy mind. After smudging a room clean, burning lavender allows you to replace the dispersed energy with warmth.

Frankincense and *myrrh* were considered to be more valuable than gold in ancient times. Used to embalm the bodies of the Egyptian pharaohs, frankincense is considered cleansing and protective of the soul. This tree resin eventually became important to most every major religion in the world and is still used in most major religious rituals. Frankincense is said to promote clairvoyance. Myrrh is a tree resin that is said to help one maintain a state of enlightenment. It also connects one to the spirit of youth and clears the path of debris that stands in the way of one's truth.

Copal is a Mexican tree sap similar to frankincense. When burned, it has a crisp, clean, sharp scent that is almost citrus-like. It is sacred to the native peoples of Mexico. Copal is the blood of trees and can be used during protection, divination, cleansing, purification, banishment, meditation, and other spiritual ceremonies. Placing small pieces of copal with your crystals and keeping them in a special place of your choice can help ward off negative energy.

Palo santo is a mystical tree that grows on the coast of South America and is related to frankincense, myrrh, and copal. *Palo santo* means "holy wood" in Spanish, and many enjoy it for its energy-cleansing and healing properties similar to those of sage and cedar. It is a strong medicine that has become popular for its heavenly presence in keeping energies grounded and clear. It provides an uplifting scent that raises one's vibration in preparation for meditation and allows for a deeper connection to the Source of all creation. It is also said that *palo santo* enhances creativity and brings good fortune to those who are open to its magic.

RITUAL
CREATE YOUR SMUDGE WAND

A sage smudge wand is wonderful to keep on hand to cleanse your own energy and to make clearance in your space.

What you will need:

Garden gloves
Fresh aromatic herbs and flowers
White sage
Scissors
Cotton string (I prefer colorful cotton thread)

Directions:

Whether you are in a garden, in an open field, or on a rooftop, take the time to be present in the space. Remove your shoes and let your feet sink into the soil if possible. Take a few breaths and listen. Walk around, observe the herbs and flowers, and consciously collect the herbs that you are most drawn to. Arrange your herbs in a bouquet with the leaves and most beautiful flowers positioned on the outside.

Starting from the bottom of the stems, wind the string around several times to bind the bundle. Trim the stems so that they are the same length and wind the string with intention around to the top, covering the leaves and blossoms and then all the way back down to the bottom, where you will wrap the string around the base and tie it in a knot, sealing in your intention. If there are any stems or flowers poking out of either end, you can trim them. Hang the wand upside down and allow it to air-dry completely for three to five days before burning it.

It's not uncommon for the smudge wand to be placed on a shell (like abalone) or on a stone, which can also be a safe space to rest it after smudging.

RITUAL
CLEARING A SPACE

These rituals will help you make space for all that is coming as you let go of the old and usher in the new.

Center yourself. Set your intention for your smudging ritual: "I drive away all stagnant energy and purify my space." Light the tip of your smudge wand and allow it to smolder. Blow onto the lit ember to help increase the rising smoke. Using your free hand, guide some smoke over your heart, holding your intention to clear energy. Start at the entrance of any room and make your way around to all corners, wafting the smoke with your hands, a fan, or a feather. Move gracefully and with intention until you have made your way back to the entrance. Open the windows and let the air flow. Play your favorite music or sit in silence in the center of the room, breathe deeply, and feel refreshed.

Smudging Yourself

Fan the swirls of smoke around your body from head to toe. You may want to focus on areas where you feel there are energetic blocks or where there has been physical, emotional, or psychic pain.

Imagine the smoke lifting away all the negative thoughts, emotions, and energies that have attached to you.

Smudging Your Purse

Perhaps you want to change your relationship with what's flowing your way financially or to attract new opportunities. If so, try a purse-smudging ritual. Empty the contents of your purse; you can do this for each one you own or just the one you are currently using. Sort through your stuff and discard what doesn't belong. Keep the remaining items neatly organized in a pile off to the side. Open the bag and take your sage and fan swirls of smoke inside and out and around the bag. By releasing and clearing the energy attached to your handbag, you are making space for what you may want to invite in. Once you finish the cleansing ritual, ground the energy you are welcoming by placing something like a new crystal or beautiful feather inside the bag. Let it air out for at least 20 minutes before you place your belongings back in.

Bag Lady

It's interesting how much we love handbags. We carry a variety of them; none of us owns just one. Some of them are gorgeous designer bags that are pretty on the outside but a total mess on the inside. Our handbags are receptacles for old and new attachments. We carry things we need on a regular basis but also things that don't belong—like old chewing gum, church candies, loose change, ticket stubs, and past receipts balled up in a bunch at the bottom of the purse. Grab your bag and turn it upside down and empty it. What's inside? Memories. Everything inside your purse has a story, and some of those objects, along with their stories, you can do without.

Your womb is like your handbag. It's in your womb space that you hold on to memories of empowerment and joy as well as the pain and trauma that are affecting your ability to create. Memories lie dormant in your cells, located in different areas of your body. In your womb, you store your memories of lovers, those with whom you have had good times and bad. The images and experiences you hold there are very real to your physical body. You need to clear away those old memories that don't serve you. When you free up the space of old memories, you make more room for new memories to form. You make space for new opportunities and keep the space clear for creativity. We'll explore that in further depth in the next portal. For now, we'll focus on clearance.

MEDITATION
WOMB CLEARANCE

Choose to sit up tall or lie flat on your back comfortably in a quiet space. Gently close your eyes. Receive three long, deep, full breaths.

Turning your vision inward, receive a deep breath in through the nose and let your internal gaze travel down to your womb. Visualize all the cords that still attach you to former partners. Visualize the cords that attach you to promises that no longer make sense for you to honor.

Exhale. Release. Identifying each cord with a former partner, thank every person for what they have taught you about yourself, then firmly cut the cord that connects you to him or her. Know that when you sever the tie, you are returning his or her energy back to that person and giving yourself permission to restore your own wholeness. Turn your attention to the promises that you have made that are keeping you from growing into your expansive potential. Cut each of those cords. Know that when you reevaluate the promises you have made and acknowledge that some simply do not work for you anymore, you have the right to release yourself of those obliga-tions. You are not beholden for the rest of your life.

Receive a deep breath in through the nose. Now exhale, sighing out through the mouth. Continue do this for each cord you visualize until all are cut. Receive a deep breath in. Now exhale. Visualize your-self pouring pure water over your womb. Water cleanses all things.

Receive a deep breath in. Now exhale. Feel refreshed and whole, ready to receive what you are now open to calling in. Allow yourself to make way for the partner your heart seeks, the project you are calling in, the baby you have been dreaming about, and the business that's in waiting. Gently open your eyes.

This is a meditation you can practice repeatedly. There are many layers to our being, and often the first time just scratches the surface.

Cleansing Our Bodies

We've done the work of clearing the space around us. I encourage you to continue—with regular meditation for womb clearance—to free yourself of memories and energies you no longer wish to carry in order to make room for what's to come. And while we've previously discussed weeding our life's garden of toxic relationships, Mother Nature's weeds—in this case, herbs—can actually *aid* in clearing the blockages of the body. What if I told you that the weeds I'm talking about can be powerful blood builders, helping to restore hormonal balance and provide a sense of rejuvenation?

Weeds are mostly misunderstood because many of us don't know what to do with them. They propagate in our gardens, outgrow the neat grass, and even rise from between the cracks in the sidewalks. Plants thriving in harsh environments are more potent and contain higher concentrations of volatile oils. Now that's what I call glow power! Look around at the ground. Powerful weeds are nestled in with other vegetation, so you may not even notice them at first glance. When I start to see a lot of dandelion and red clover bunches in nature, I know it's time to collect these plants and do my own internal spring cleaning. Could something growing from the sidewalk cracks be good for you? Think of them as Mother Nature's first line of defense. You can start by trying herbal teas such as dandelion, nettle, yarrow, ginger, or red clover.

Wise Weeds: Our Herbal Allies

Dandelion: With a name meaning "lion's tooth" in French, dandelion is rich in vitamins A and C, iron, and calcium. It is detoxifying, which explains why it's included in many medicines. Its high levels of dietary fiber make it a beneficial aid for digestion and proper intestinal health. Dietary fiber stimulates regular, healthy bowel movements by adding bulk to our stool. Dandelion is a strong, bitter herb that has an astringent and cleansing effect on the liver and kidneys. It helps to break down fats stored in the liver and gallbladder and promotes healthy colon function. It's a great plant to introduce when we transition from eating hearty winter foods to light, spring-inspired meals. The young leaves are a great addition to sandwiches. You can also add dandelion greens to a mixed-green salad. To pack in extra protein, add some raw pumpkin seeds, hemp seeds, or walnuts. Sprinkle in some highly mineralized dulse seaweed flakes, and add some avocado slices and your favorite salad dressing, and you're in business.

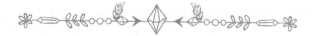

SAUTEED DANDELION GREENS WITH GARLIC

(NOTE: please buy organically grown dandelion. Since most folks consider them a pesky weed, when they are found in nature, they have often been heavily sprayed.)

2 lbs dandelion greens, thoroughly washed
2 tbsp olive oil
5 cloves garlic, bruised and smashed open
crushed red pepper and sea salt to taste

Blanch the greens in salted water for up to 60 seconds. Then shock the greens in a bowl of ice water to stop them from cooking and to retain the green color. Drain and lightly squeeze out water. Heat the oil in a skillet, then add the garlic, cooking over medium-low heat. As the garlic begins to brown, add in the greens and stir to coat them in the garlicky oil. Cover and raise the heat to medium high. Cook for an additional 3 minutes. Season with sea salt and crushed red pepper.

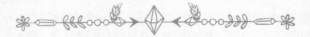

Nettles: Highly nutritious stinging nettles are a prickly plant often used as a spring tonic. They're a natural detoxifier that removes metabolic waste and are both gentle and stimulating on the lymphatic system, promoting easy excretion through the kidneys. Stinging nettles reduce PMS symptoms, process estrogen to relieve menopausal symptoms, and curb excess menstrual flow. They're often used in herbal tonics to remove fibroids and regulate menstrual flow. Nettles destroy intestinal worms and parasites and support the endocrine system, including the thyroid, spleen, and pancreas.

Yarrow: Yarrow is such a wonderful womb-working herb for the reproductive system; it can both quell heavy bleeding and stimulate bleeding if it is scant. It also works to eliminate the congestion that results in dark, clotted blood and period pains. It is useful for vaginal infections or irregular discharge as well as spotting between periods. Yarrow is a great urinary antiseptic. Drink as a warm or cool infusion to remedy cystitis and urinary-tract infections.

Ginger: The pungent ingredient of ginger, found in Asian and Caribbean-inspired meals, packs a lot more punch than just flavor. Ginger acts as a cleansing agent for the bowels, kidneys, and skin, is soothing for the stomach, and is effective for fighting off colds. Ginger improves circulation throughout the tissues and is excellent for the respiratory system by aiding in the expansion of your lungs and the loosening of phlegm. It is a natural expectorant that breaks down and removes mucus from the body. This great-tasting herb is famous for its amazing digestive benefits. Grate it into soups, stir-fries, and marinades for a powerful health boost.

Red clover: Considered one of the richest sources of isoflavones (water-soluble chemicals that act like estrogens and are found in many plants), red clover is used for hot flashes/flushes, lowering cholesterol, breast enhancement and breast health, improving urine production, and improving circulation of the blood. It is also used to help prevent osteoporosis and to reduce the possibility of blood clots and arterial plaques. Red clover is often taken to relieve symptoms of PMS like breast tenderness. It also works against uterine fibroids.

For a gentle, cleansing herbal tea, try the red clover recipe below. You can find organic red clover blossoms at herbal shops, farmers' markets, and online. Or, if you take the time to wander through some blossoming fields outside the city limits, you can harvest bundles of this herb yourself. For an even more potent womb-clearing mixture, add nettles, either ½ cup fresh or ¼ cup dried.

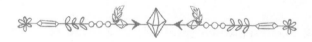

RED CLOVER HERBAL TEA

1 cup fresh red clover blossoms (or ½ cup dried)
¼ cup fresh mint leaves
4 cups filtered water
agave nectar to taste

Bring water to a boil. Add clover blossoms and mint. Allow to steep up to 10 minutes. Strain off the liquid and sweeten if desired.

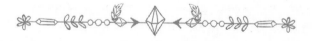

RITUAL
RELEASING CEREMONY

All the work we have done up to this moment has been about uncovering and exploring what holds us back to make space for what we are calling in. Clearing the physical spaces in our lives and our bodies and weeding out our relationships may be emotionally trying but feels grounding. This exercise is an opportunity to give concrete physical action to the way we release our emotional baggage.

What you will need:

> 2 sheets of paper
> a pen
> a highlighter
> white sage smudging wand
> matches

Work this ritual when you have at least 30 to 40 minutes of uninterrupted time. On one sheet of paper, make two columns. In the first, write out the things you are ready to release today. Be as descriptive as possible. In the second column, write down the things you want to release but need to work up the courage to let go of. Write down why you feel attached to the things in this column.

On your next sheet of paper, make two columns. At the top of the first column, write "I release" and at the top of the second, "I embrace." In the release column, write down everything you are letting go of—resentment of an ex, hatred of your boss, your mother's expectations of you, your self-attacking. In the embrace column, list the steps you will take to go deeper into those issues you are not yet willing to release—getting a therapist to talk through some of the challenges, seeking out a spiritual advisor or coach, meditating or praying more, surrounding yourself with supportive friends.

The final step will be to rip up the paper (you can burn it if you wish) and smudge yourself. First, find a comfortable area to situate yourself in. Light one end of the smudge wand until the smoke begins to come forth. Waving the tip with the lit ember will create even more smoke. We create a smoky environment with incense because it's the medium that spirits breathe in.

As you swirl the smudge wand around, start to recite the statements out loud from each column—"I release my resentment of my ex," "I embrace love and joy entering my life." Move through everything on your lists. Then sit still for about 5 to 10 minutes with your eyes closed for a meditation. Just receive, inhaling peace and serenity and exhaling stress and anxiety. Tear up the paper and, if you feel comfortable doing so, burn it safely outside.

Now that you have released some emotional baggage, return to your journal and write down three commitments you may take toward nurturing yourself, the timeline for implementation, and how you will make these new commitments into new practices. Write down what support is necessary to help yourself succeed and move forward.

New You

Do you want to be a vessel for creativity and an overflowing fountain of abundance? Do you want to attract love into your life? Are you itching to discover a new facet of yourself? We simply cannot continue to invest energy into our superficial neuroses, dramas, resentments, or fears and yet claim to be a space for creativity, abundance, and love. It's time to surrender those things that do not lead us to the highest good; they are blocking us from the magic within and the incredible ride of living in joy. In order for there to be flow, we must surrender, not because we are attached to a particular outcome but because it is the right choice—the only choice.

How many conferences or retreats have you attended, feeling high on life, only to return to your habitual patterns when that inspiration fizzles? How many times have you told yourself, "I'm gonna leave this job," "I'm gonna break up with this person," "I'm ready for change," and a few days later, you are back in your regular groove, comfortable again with the subpar arrangement you have relegated yourself to? You must be willing to give up the cushy job for the possibility of building the business of your dreams. You must release the dysfunctional relationship and risk being alone rather than stay and compromise your happiness and potential for fulfillment of love. When you set the deepest intentions for your life, you need to consciously align your thoughts and actions with them, so check your alignment. You deserve all the goodness coming your way—tap into your GPS and stay ready to receive.

Your Personal Mission

What we're working toward together is helping you live your best life by calling for and welcoming change for yourself. Now that we've made some space and taken the time to engage with your intuition, let's connect you with what you truly value. It's time to write down for yourself exactly what you're seeking. Is it a new relationship? Is it a new job? Is it a healthier body? Whatever it is, this is your current personal mission. This is your seed goal unfolded. We may take this journey together and then come out on the other side ready to start again with a new goal, on a new path. And at that time, we'll rewrite our personal mission statement and start again, in an ever-turning cycle of creating and attuning to our best self.

After tuning in to your GPS and taking some time for reflection, you should have some more clarity about what is calling to you at this time, about the transformative journey you set out on in order to create your best life. It's your divine responsibility to become the best iteration of yourself and bring all your passion and gifts to the world during this lifetime. Your life is worth a noble mission, so seek to unfold it. Remember that your life is a sacred record of time, and you will never have more time than you do right now. Draft your **personal mission statement.** It's only for you to see, but it's something to reference and keep you on track. I'm going to give four questions to get you started:

> What do I feel called to change in my life right now?
>
> What inspires me more than anything else?
>
> What dream, desire, activity, or service am I being guided to pursue?

Where will I find the inspiration to make that change?

How can practicing vulnerability help me achieve my mission?

Name your intention:

Give one example of how you will prioritize yourself to target your personal mission.

Give one affirmation that will help you keep a positive focus and remain inspired and on track with your personal mission.

Whatever you answered here is what you were put here to spend your time doing. The sky is not the limit; it's the view. It's scary to take the journey sometimes, but know that everyone who ever made something remarkable of themselves started someplace small and trusted their crazy, creative idea.

We are all divine works in progress. Constantly align your daily choices with the goal or outcome you want to achieve. Just focus on following your creative mandate and fulfilling your vision. That sends a message to the Universe that you are clear, you are ready, and you have unshakable faith and patience. You will be rewarded with miracles that affirm that you are on the right path. Stay on mission. That is the path to ultimate freedom.

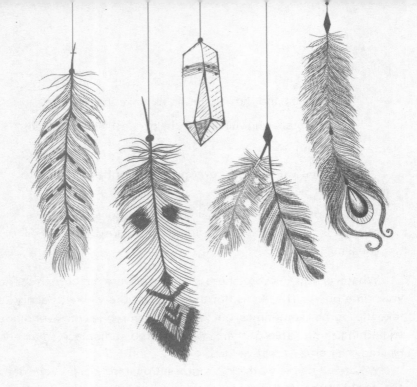

*"And the day came when the risk
to remain tight in a bud was more painful
than the risk it took to blossom."*

- Anaïs Nin

MOTIVATION MIX TRACK
"FREEDOM" by Beyoncé, *Lemonade*

portal no. 2

IGNITE

ignite |ig′ nī t|
verb: to catch fire or cause to catch fire
• to arouse or inflame (an emotion or situation)

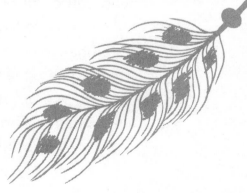

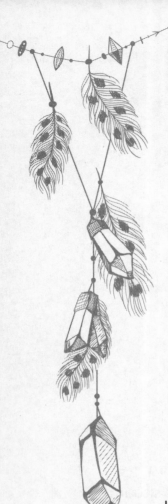

INVOCATION

~

Soften into Deep Listening
Awareness
Candles Flickering
Evanescent warmth
Fills the space
The seraphic feminine
Awakened
Air dense
Perfumed by Palo Santo
And sanctified fantasies
Magnolia flower offering
At the altar of my soul
Loved etched upon my wounds
We are Whole
Inhale rolling waves
Exhale ocean spray
We breathe
Open palmed and anointed
With gratitude
We Receive

~

spirituality and contemplative practice

"Enlightened leadership is spiritual if we understand spirituality not as some kind of religious dogma or ideology but as the domain of awareness where we experience values like truth, goodness, beauty, love and compassion, and also intuition, creativity, insight and focused attention."

~ DEEPAK CHOPRA

It's time to explore spirituality—our relationship to the Divine. Spiritual practice is a crucial element in enhancing your glow power, standing in your purpose and stirring up feminine forces to create a vacuum attracting what you want most. We've already uncovered our blocks and cleared the space for our intentions to evoke our deep desires. We will call upon God, the benevolent Universe, Consciousness, the Most High, or Spirit to be a guiding and restorative force as we ready ourselves to step out onto the path to come.

Spiritual practice—formal or informal—is such an important part of preparing yourself for a transformative journey. A spiritual practice provides us with fortitude and gratitude for whatever comes our way. My relationship to Spirit fuels me up. It gives me the energy and the confidence to move forward and improves my ability to withstand and bounce back from the challenges I face on my journey. It's a bridge to self-awareness and provides a space to go within myself to surrender and find grounding. Spirituality is a tool for actualizing my best self, putting my energy into drawing out that best self, and is the way I connect to what's *bigger* than myself. That connection allows me to keep perspective on my own journey in the context of the larger universe. It helps me to stay tapped into my GPS, which is a gift from God.

Your relationship with the cosmic power, God, and the infinite is an important part of owning your glow. A reflective practice is a gateway to fine-tuning your GPS. When you believe that you are protected and guided, that the glory lies in following the internal light that's beaming through you, you can do anything. When we consciously connect with spirit, we are reminded that our life has a bigger purpose and is much more than the sum of our problems. Daily prayer, Sunday services, Shabbat dinner, meditation, chanting, soul singing, hiking in nature, working it out on a yoga mat—however you feel most authentic engaging with the Divine is your way of being in presence with that power. If it centers your being in oneness with spirit, then it works. What keeps you spiritually grounded?

Building Your Spiritual Self-Confidence

Incorporating a spiritual practice into your life doesn't require a rummage sale of your flyest stilettos to trade in for Birkenstocks and *nag champa* incense. It doesn't mean you have to wear holy robes and abstain from life's sweetness. It doesn't mean you can't rock a turban, *mala* beads, *and* a Céline bag all at the same time. It does not require you to cut off any part of who you are to show up for the party within. It simply requires you to show up. You might be new to these ideas, and it may even be uncomfortable to talk about Spirit, God, or the angels, but you will eventually find the spiritual lexicon that jibes with your story and your lifestyle.

I grew up in a Catholic household with my mother and attended Catholic grammar school. I went to Mass with my grandmother, a devout Catholic, and although I felt a strong connection with my faith, it didn't seem celebratory enough for me. While others found solace or joy in the services, I always walked away the idea that I should apologize for who I was. The focus, for me, of the Catholic faith was on sin, and that didn't speak to what I was looking for spiritually. What worked for my grandmother, I learned, didn't suit my personality or my outlook on life. When I visited my father in Southern California, though, I would go to an A.M.E. (African Methodist Episcopal) church. It was a black church where the women would wear huge hats and carry fans to keep cool in the pews. The old ladies would rock back and forth and lift their hands up toward the heavens, eyes closed in grace, and shout *"Glory, glory!"* in the name of Jesus. The congregation was lively and praised the Lord out loud. Now this was a soulful type of service I could get down with! I loved the energy, the gospel-music ministry—they lit up every cell in my body through praise. I had never felt anything dance in my heart the way the sound of the organ, piano, and choir all harmonizing together did. I joined the choir because it lifted my spirit and gave me a sense of belonging.

As a little girl, my spiritual awakening was not traditional. I was also deeply enchanted by nature, and so that became my religion as well. I saw God in every living thing—every butterfly, every flower, every puppy, every ant, every tree, and every spider. Well, maybe not the spiders. But I believed in the church of Mother Nature, and following her path was abiding by her rhythms—observing moon cycles, respecting and yielding to the seasons, and having reverence for her creations—plants and animals. I went on to learn about divination practices that also revere Nature and personify natural forces, from Vedic astrology to the Native American traditions of the Nez Perce and Cherokee.

As an adult, particularly around the time of my pregnancy, I became enchanted by the goddesses of different global cultures, particularly the Hindu Triple Goddess archetype (Lakshmi, Durga, and Saraswati) and the goddesses Yemaya and Oshun from the West African Yoruba tradition. I loved the stories of folklore and how they drove the Gods crazy with their whims. I danced Afro-Cuban and performed Afro-Brazilian dance and learned the sequences for each prominent deity. And when I lived in Brazil in the early 2000s, in the spiritual houses of *Candomblé,* I experienced firsthand female priests being venerated above the men and the cultural impact that powerful female deities had on society.

At New Year's, when people are usually out partying, the Cariocas—residents of Rio de Janeiro—bring an offering to the goddess Iemanjá (same as the aforementioned Yemaya), the ruler and protector of the seawaters. They dress in all white to signify cleansing and renewal and pay respects at the edge of the water with white flowers, candles, rice, and perfume. The sea is life in Brazil, and Iemanjá is the crowned queen. She is associated with fertility and prosperity, children, birthing, the home, and family. She is the merciful goddess of creation and protector of women during conception and childbirth, as well as of children. She is a deep ocean of comfort for those in need. Legend says that one might send out prayers on the water on little rafts for her to answer. I felt completely aligned with the legend of Goddess Iemanjá, powerful and undoubtedly firm in her femininity.

All these interests, intrigues, and colorful spiritual experiences at home and abroad shaped my view of religion and the spirit realm. They gave me a sense of where I see myself in the world and where I place and value the unseen. Rather than denounce things that weren't a part of the religious tradition that I was born into, I embraced what I found to be fulfilling spiritually. I pulled them into my practice and rituals because spirituality is agile and inclusive. I gathered found objects that reminded me of the goddesses and placed them upon my altars. I incorporated them into my yoga practice as well.

There are no boundaries when it comes to spirit. It's about what moves you, what takes you higher. The only criterion is that you embrace what makes you feel at home. When I am soul-clapping in a Baptist church and singing at the top of my lungs, I feel at home. When I am placing a bed of white flowers on the water as an offering to Iemanjá, I feel at home. When I am spreading into a warrior II pose on my yoga mat, I feel at home. When I am walking barefoot in the woods and picking dandelions, I feel at home. When I am swaying my hips in darkness and singing along to Solange, I feel at home. When I am lying in bed next to my beloved, gazing into his eyes, I feel at home. When I am alone, I still feel at home. That ability to feel at home wherever you are is what spiritual self-confidence is all about.

Many of us never feel at home, because we aren't at home in our own bodies. All the places you've been taught to be afraid of—to discard—are where you find your glow power. All the parts you are shaming, cursing, and wishing away—those that are intrinsically feminine—are the key to your personal power. If you knew it, you would be unstoppable.

YOUR POWER IS NOT FOR SOMEONE TO HAND OVER TO YOU BUT FOR YOU TO SEEK AND RECLAIM FOR YOURSELF.

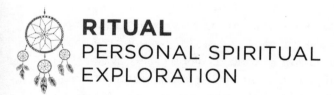

RITUAL
PERSONAL SPIRITUAL EXPLORATION

Spiritual guidance is always available to you. As you deepen your tether to this force, you will be able to see the signs laid out before you and tap into the reservoir of the Divine.

Answer these questions in your journal and reflect on how the information you uncover might help you move forward toward stronger spiritual self-confidence and better spiritual self-awareness.

What was your spiritual upbringing?

What elements of that spiritual upbringing still speak to you?

Are there elements of that spiritual upbringing that you wish to leave behind?

What spiritual practices are you drawn to that resonate with you?

How comfortable are you with organized religion?

Are you comfortable sharing your spirituality with others, or is it a more private endeavor?

Do you feel anchored in a spiritual community?

What are your experiences with or thoughts about traditional prayer?

Do you have someone in your life who actively supports you in your spiritual growth? If not, whom do you know who might fill that role?

Discovering Your Spiritual Path

Are you still unsure about exactly what your own spiritual practice should look like? Just as I have, you too can explore all the spiritual possibilities on offer. There are many avenues for exploring religious and spiritual practices: taking a world-religions class, revisiting a religious practice you might have left behind in your youth, attending services with a willing friend of a different religion, attending a shamanic ceremony, reading holy texts, joining a prayer circle, joining a faith-based group online to engage in spiritual discourse, attending a mindfulness class, gathering at a women's circle, attending local services when you travel, and exploring local traditions. There is an important aspect to spirituality that has less to do with mainstream religion or cultural traditions and teachings and more to do with stillness.

Stillness and Soul

An important step on this journey is to integrate a spiritual practice into your life that includes being still. Stillness is a contemplative practice that allows us to experience moments of clarity and helps us stay attuned to our GPS. When you are still, it doesn't mean you are doing nothing, but that you can feel all that is happening through you because you are dialed in. We practice stillness by incorporating meditation. Meditation is a practice that expands our consciousness. Usually practiced seated, meditation allows us to slow down and be present with ourselves. The numerous health benefits include stress reduction, improved mood, increased self-esteem, increased sense of joy and compassion, and an improved sense of overall well-being. Meditation boosts the immune system because it helps to combat the effect of stress hormones on our nervous system. Meditation is deep listening. It's a practice that can lead to a mindful life.

Mindfulness is not the same thing as meditation, although we achieve mindfulness *through* meditation. Mindfulness is a state of active, open attention and a growing awareness of self and your environment. Mindfulness is expanding into awareness and compassion, acceptance of and kindness to yourself, others, and the world. Through mindfulness we can begin to let go of our attachment to what we think we should be doing and move toward acceptance of what is happening in the present moment.

Mindfulness helps you focus your energy and induces a state of calm. It can completely transform your life, making you aware of your emotions and physical and emotional reactions. Practice makes for progress, and getting comfortable with your meditation practice is contingent on doing it regularly. Start small and build from there. Let your body guide you into a practice of 10 minutes a day to start, using one of the many meditation apps with which you can set a timer. Sit and breathe and repeat the mantra: *In this present moment, all is well.*

If this is somewhat new for you, here's how you can incorporate both meditation and mindfulness into your spiritual practice. You might find it helpful to join a meditation studio or take an intro course. You can also download apps like Headspace, Inscape, or Insight Timer that will modulate the process of meditation for you.

Get a nice pillow or meditation cushion and set aside a space in your home or workspace where you can sit in silence. You may find music helpful in keeping you engaged as you get more comfortable, or the ambient sounds of your surroundings may be stimulating enough. I encourage a regular practice of sitting where you are, immersing yourself in those sounds. I also find recorded crystal sound bowls incredibly neutralizing. Sitting outside in nature can be a great way to anchor your practice. You may be only one step away from a full-blown meditation practice if you're already practicing yoga but haven't quite moved beyond just the physical part of it.

Incorporating Spiritual Practice into Your Life

Now that you've made it through the work of discovering what spiritual practices you're most comfortable with, it's time to do the work of incorporating them into your day.

You are the beginning of a movement. It's about birthing yourself. Your soul flashlight shines your glow power. The way you make this spiritual practice a part of your daily life is to take a few minutes a day and just do it. Below we'll explore several methods of making Spirit a part of your life, but there is no preset road map. You are building a framework from scratch. There is no one right way; there is your way. So, go and forge it. Be the little ripple that grows into a wave. Pay attention to synchronistic signs and symbology in your daily life because that's one of the ways Spirit speaks to us. Are there patterns, numbers, repetition, an awakening? These moments are valid and often signals that we are attuned to our path.

Observe Your Sabbath

Traditionally speaking, the Sabbath is a day of rest. It's a time to reconnect to the sacred in your life and give thanks. You might attend weekly church or temple services or perhaps spend time in nature as your source of renewal. Whatever your divine practice, choose a day to hold your own Sabbath. It may not be on Saturday or Sunday; it may not even be an all-day ritual. If your schedule absolutely does not allow for a weekly Sabbath, you might choose a few hours each day or even a few minutes each day at the bare minimum.

This is a time to unplug from work and routine, a time to disconnect with the outer world and slow your pace, to enjoy family and time alone. Take time to walk outside. Cook a slow meal and savor it with gratitude. Relax with a candlelit bath and a good book. Write poetry. Get a massage and don't check your phone afterward; just be. What are the many ways you can pour back into yourself? What's your ritual for giving thanks? What helps to dial you back into what's important and what's holy? This Sabbath observance is at the essence of what I call *glow time.* It is all about honoring the Divine within and creating sacred portals of self-renewal.

Creating Your Own Altar

Altars are energetically charged, sacred spaces for ritual. They are not relegated to churches. When I was in India, altars were everywhere—in the streets, under trees, and in other unexpected places outside of temples. I was so moved by these public displays of devotion. You can turn any surface into an altar. It can be as simple as placing objects on a table or shelf that remind you of important people and events in your life. With thoughtfulness, you can transform any space into a sacred sanctuary.

I've gathered objects from around the world and used them to create altar spaces that hold the energy that I want to cultivate in my personal space and in my life. You can collect beautiful glass vases, flowers, sculptures, talismans, seashells, rocks, gemstones, or crystals and place them on your altar. Photographs of elders, leaders, figures from history, or goddesses that inspire you should be placed upon the altar for tribute and to evoke the energy of encouragement. Consider which colors bring you joy, peace, and tranquility. Begin to adorn your altar and let your GPS guide you. Once you complete it, you can update it frequently with new items and swap pictures, candles, and colors as well.

Take the time to sit before your altar daily for prayer or meditation focused on those aspects of your life that bring you comfort and happiness. If you're someone who travels often, you can take your altar elements with you and set up an altar wherever you are.

Establish a Regular Meditation/Prayer Practice

Spiritual fitness is a gift. Are you feeling spiritually fit? Jesus said, "The kingdom of God is within you." And meditation teaches us to focus our attention inward, relax the body, and observe the breath while quieting the mind, thus opening us up to receiving more guidance. Meditation also increases our awareness and heightens our senses. We become keenly aware of everything happening around us. Your relationship to the Divine is ever evolving. A benevolent force within and surrounding you is guiding you along your path. Your GPS is a direct line to Spirit. Prayer is also a powerful way to connect with Spirit. Where meditation is a process of listening and receiving, prayer is a process of petitioning and thanking. You can pray in any way you feel comfortable with.

Find a sacred space in your home, whether at the altar you've set up or some other private spot, where you can sit in silence and tune inward. Deep breathing and focused concentration slow down brain waves, making them more organized. This allows us to activate the parasympathetic nervous system, releasing endorphins into the bloodstream and allowing the brain to emit only happy hormones! This helps us to have presence, peace of mind, and maintain a practice of gratitude. If giving thanks is a part of your practice, your inner light will shine! I am always so amazed at what comes my way when I count my blessings.

"*The more you praise and celebrate your life, the more there is in life to celebrate.*"

- Oprah Winfrey

MEDITATION
BAREFOOT GROUNDING

This meditation requires you to go outside. Whether you are in the city or the countryside, I want you to find yourself on terra firma in a garden, city park, or backyard. Stand on solid Mother Earth, in your bare feet. Our bodies are bioelectrical in nature. The functions of our cells and nervous system are governed by electrical power and pulses of energy. Electrons and fluids in Earth's core generate continuous, powerful magnetic forces and complex energy fields. Earth's energetic cycles and rhythms play important roles in our bodies' electrical rhythms, such as regulation of our hormone production and sleep-wake cycles.

Barefoot grounding can help relieve chronic pain, reduce stress and anxiety, and improve sleep. Damp soil is more conductive and can accelerate the benefits of grounding. The benefits are cumulative, so make this meditation a ritual practice. Do this in the daytime when the sun has warmed up the earth. As the sunlight kisses your face, gently close your eyes.

Receive a full belly breath and exhale, and ground your feet firmly into the soil. Wiggle your toes and sink your feet more deeply into the earth. Inhale the serenity of the outdoors, and exhale tension. Inhale awe, and exhale stress or anxiety. Each day brings awe, wonder, and gratitude. You nurture your soul in tune with the living energy universe, cultivating a beautiful life. You honor the healthy body you live within and are grateful for the miracle of life. You experience the sacred in all things as you create your own sanctuary for renewal, walking through the garden gate to enter the portal of the Divine. Here you are deeply nurtured as you feel connected to all creation. How awakened are you to the dancing Universe and your own internal dance? The precious gifts of sunlight, warmth, the beauty of flowers, and the vastness of the stars above envelop you in the mysterious. You celebrate the blossoms and the harvest and find yourself pulsing within the rhythms of nature. Listen to the music of the ambient landscape, Mother Nature's sacred sound. Receive a breath and take your arms up and overhead, and exhale with your palms together in prayer position. When you are ready, gently open your eyes.

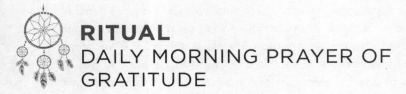

RITUAL
DAILY MORNING PRAYER OF GRATITUDE

Bring the power of prayer into your morning. Make this a daily ritual. Each morning before you get up and moving, place one hand on your heart and one on your belly and breathe deeply. Look out the window and toward the sky. Embrace yourself and speak a prayer of gratitude and ask Spirit for any clarity or guidance.

Thank you for waking me up today. Thank you for protecting and watching over me. I am well in spirit and mind and capable of greatness. May I walk in the path of my highest self and be present to the beauty, blessing, and abundance you provide. Please order my steps and guide me to the places I need to be and toward the people I need to see. Touch everything in my life with your holy hand and make me a vessel for your will. I am so thankful, so joyful. Thank you.

Come up with your own morning prayers. Reach over to your journal to write down a minimum of three things you are grateful for. To thrive, we must honor and protect our sacredness. Each day, care for the temple that houses your spirit and is the seat and power of your thought, wisdom, and creativity.

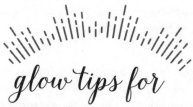

glow tips for
Building Spirituality Into Your Daily Life

Read spiritual texts. Find a spiritual or inspirational text, scripture, or poetry to dive into first thing in the morning to start your day on a positive track and keep you tapped into greatness.

Get stoned. I don't mean do drugs! I mean get adorned with crystals, gemstones, *malas*, and more. *Malas* are meditation garlands that have been used for thousands of years by spiritual seekers around the world. Like rosary beads, they are an ancient tool for prayer. Both *malas* and rosaries can also be worn for their properties and meaning. *Mala* beads can be used in a variety of ways to help you achieve your dreams and desires. Start by using your *mala* with intention or associating it with a particular mantra, prayer, or sound. Wear it around your neck or clasp it firmly in your palms as you tune in and focus on your breath. I wear my *mala* beads when I travel and use them for prayer before I take off for a flight. You can also bring your beads to your mat during your yoga practice as a way to focus and bring awareness to your intentions, infusing your mala with the energy of your practice.

Embrace sacred objects. There are symbols and meanings in sacred objects, and they can be powerful tools for awakening your latent spiritual life. Angels, candles, feathers, crystals, buddhas, and more are all symbolic objects that you should place on your desk, in your car, or at your altar at home.

Craft your own affirmations. Make a daily habit of coming up with your own affirmations. The godmother of affirmations, Louise Hay, founder of Hay House, shares her affirmations with the world every day via social media.

Listen to uplifting music. This includes podcasts as well. Rather than the news, put on devotional music for serenity or gospel and be joyful.

Get outside. Take a walk in nature and honor the beauty surrounding you. Feel gratitude for it. Reflect on the intricacies found within it. How blessed and sacred is nature! Even in the most concrete of jungles, beauty can be found everywhere.

Make a God box. Craft a God box from an oatmeal box or tin that you fashion with collage elements. Cut a slit in the top of the box. When you have a prayer or an intention, write it down, fold it up, and place it inside the God box. It can live at your altar.

Find a spiritual community or home. Whether it's a house of worship, a group-coaching community, a meditation or women's circle, or a yoga class, find a community that will support you in your quest for personal and spiritual growth. It will enhance every aspect of your life. Sometimes the people closest to us aren't the best ones to take the journey with; they may not yet understand our path. Finding a sympathetic spiritual community is key to building your support network.

Practice moon mapping. Plan your calendar in alignment with the lunar phases, primarily new moon and full moon to start. Plan rituals for the new moon, whose energy is associated with beginnings and planting seeds. Create rituals for the full moon, whose energy is aligned with completion and harvest.

Eat, pray, glow. Plan a spiritual quest. Choose a place with symbolic significance. Perhaps it's a place that has been on your mood board for a while, or it's a place you've always wanted to visit. Go for your own personal development, alone or in a group. I went to India, and this experience for me was profound and deeply spiritual.

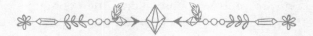

Acknowledging Your Ancestral Guides

Our ancestors are our biggest allies. One of the most sacred gifts we can offer our ancestors is fulfilling our life's calling. When we live out our potential, we honor the path and legacy we come from. Remember your loved ones who are no longer with us and who are now in the spirit realm. Remember the ancestors and stories that shape your unique history. Honor the lineage of powerful women who came before you. Elevate your ancestors in candlelight. Always acknowledge the spirits and elders who have paved the way for you, and they will help you accomplish your goals in life. You may feel a magnetic connection to ancestral lineage other than your own. Light a candle weekly, as it will bring spiritual light into your home. Light your incense of choice. My grandmother says, "Incense is the medium that spirits breathe in." Invite them in to breathe with you. What have you inherited from your ancestry that needs healing? What valuable magic has been passed down to you that needs to be activated?

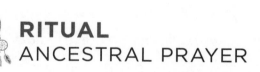

RITUAL
ANCESTRAL PRAYER

Light a candle and sit in silence. Ask for guidance as you tune in to the silence. Start to speak to your ancestors silently or out loud.

I honor my unique gifts, talents, and powers. I come from a strong and powerful people.

I release the baggage and ancestral wounds that have been passed on to me. I will turn the pain and struggle of my past into purpose. I celebrate the freedom that I have because of sacrifices made before me. I promise to honor my lineage and live out my truth.

I bow to the legacy that gave rise to me. Through my thoughts and actions, I pave the path for a legacy I will leave behind.

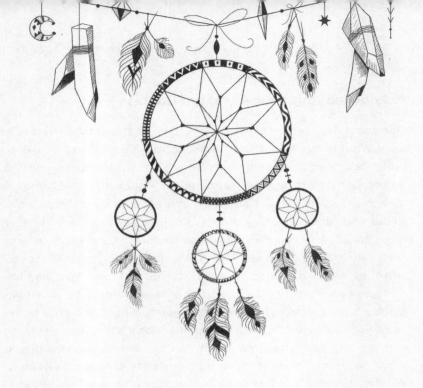

"*Spirituality can release blocks, lead you to ideas, and make your life artful. Sometimes when we pray for guidance, we're guided in unexpected directions. We may want a lofty answer and we get the intuition to clean our bedroom.*"

- Julia Cameron

feminine forces: wombifesting and sacred cycles

"You're on this earth with a divine purpose: to rise to the level of your highest creative possibility, expressing all that you are intellectually, emotionally, psychologically, and physically in order to make the universe a more beautiful place."

~ MARIANNE WILLIAMSON

Creativity comes from one place—from within us. Anything we wish to bring forth is spawned in our wombs and cultivated until it's time to yield the fruits to the world. Like in an anatomical pregnancy—where a child grows within the uterus, creating expansion, growth in consciousness, increased awareness, strength, courage, and infinite possibility—our ideas gestate. They start miniscule, like an egg at the point of fertilization, then begin a process of proliferation. The idea grows when you speak it, share it, get input, write it down, and develop strategy around it. You then grow your concept into a vision that is executed in the world. It becomes something tangible—a screenplay, a business plan, a choreographed dance, a book, a new product offering, a solution to a problem. Even when you aren't directly working on it, it's still taking shape. Just as a mother can be sitting still while metabolic and catabolic processes are underway, creating the very tissues that will result in a perfect human baby, you are cultivating your vision even when you are asleep or meditating. When you are still, you create space for more opening, heightened awareness, and the ever-so-sweet aha moments that become more and more frequent.

The womb is receptive, soft, and a container for cultivation. And the act of creating something from that place, of accessing our womb space and drawing to us that which we most desire, is called wombifestation. It's the opposite of the *manifesting* power that so many modern spiritual leaders and thought-leaders talk about. Manifestation has become correlated with "making it happen," whereas *wombifesting* is "letting it happen." It's a fierce allowance, saying yes to what you want and letting it come, whether it's a job, a romantic partner, a new car, a baby—it's whatever you are dreaming of, envisioning, and holding space for. See, there is tremendous value in being a go-getter, getting things done, making shit happen, and we as women are very skilled in this arena. There are qualities within us that we should enhance by also acknowledging the uniquely *feminine* force of receptivity. Men and women are both good at making shit happen, but we have this other force working in our favor, and we should play to that. I'd like to note that you don't have to have been born with a uterus or currently have one to embrace this concept. There is power in the dynamic force of wombifesting, fluid energy in allowance and receptivity, of setting an intention, cultivating awareness, and allowing something to show up. That feminine force is magic, and employing it is a powerful way to walk through life. It is the magic of owning your glow.

I used to be surprised when something on my vision board occurred in my waking reality. Then I realized that it wasn't just happening *to* me, it was happening *through* me. I had put it there. I had placed these dreams and desired experiences within my mind as aspirations. The dreams came to life when the time and circumstances were ripe, not when I desired. Not when it was convenient for me or my ego, but when I had done the work and was ready to fully embody what it meant to be in that moment that I aspired to. When the circumstances were ready to support me and when I was fully ready to be supported—felt *worthy* of that experience—was when it miraculously appeared in my life. People always ask, "How do you know when it's your time?" You will know because it will feel effortless. When the Universe knows you are ready, it will swan-dive into your life with everything you need to take the first step.

I am not simply advocating for you to pray for what you want, kick back and relax, and expect that you will get it. "The Universe will provide" philosophy has been misapplied by many who believe that you can simply ask for what you want and it will be handed to you, with no work involved. My philosophy is much more dynamic than that. It's not a complacent process. You can't be lazy when you want something; you must do the work for it, too. Being receptive is an active state of being. In nature, the spider makes weaving her web a meditation and focuses on creating a vortex of energy that draws the prey to her. She doesn't go out to hunt it. She dwells in the certainty that when she does her part, Mother Nature does the rest, and food is provided. Observe how flowers use their beauty and fragrant scent to seduce the pollinators. Flowers can't pull up their roots and go proliferate on their own. They depend on the insects and animals to help spread their pollen, so they use stillness to create an energy vacuum to draw the bees, birds, and butterflies.

Have you ever been so laser-focused on something, yet it seems to elude you? And then, once you forget about it and focus on what you're doing, it seems to find its way back into your orbit, seemingly by design. Do you think that is a coincidence?

Like most feminine processes, *letting it happen* is powerful, and yet it is seen as a form of weakness. In a culture obsessed with conquest and control, we've forgotten the very basics when it comes to attraction. When you let it happen, you, my dear, are at the helm. You choose, you summon it, you invite it forth, you stir the pot, you make the space for it—so that instead of spending energy actively hustling and pursuing the desired outcome, you dream it, hold space for it, and draw it near. The vision blooms within you and becomes reality. Like a spider with her web, you create the very vacuum that invites the opportunity to occur.

We'll locate the center of all our creativity in the womb, learn to slow down in order to allow for wombifestation, explore the two major forces—lunar cycles and menstrual cycles—that act upon our bodies and influence the womb space, and discuss how they intersect and how we can align with them to create space for what we want. We are moving from the "Evoke" portal where we were calling and summoning forth our creative prowess to the "Ignite" portal where we are lighting up the fire. We're going from discovering what we want to call to us to actively placing that call. Wombifesting is the process of allowing our dreams to come into reality. Let's light it up!

A Need to Create

I once had a client who suffered mild reproductive-health issues. She wanted to have a baby. She also really wanted a thriving career as a writer but spent too much of her creative energy focused on her day job, real estate, which she was admittedly good at. She could move a Manhattan apartment on Park Avenue with her eyes closed. She had money—lots of it. She had help—lots of it—trainers, acupuncturists, crystal healers, therapists . . . she was surrounded by light-workers, but no one offered her the guidance or advice she needed. You see, Erica was driven, focused, determined to build the dream that her parents wanted her to have, to make money for a company she didn't believe in, to sustain a life that she didn't love. She was in crisis.

Her boss had become concerned with her performance. The anxiety to perform under pressure was causing Erica to crack, because she didn't have healthy outlets in place. She didn't have her writing to retreat to. She was never in the mood for sex, because she was so irritable about work and lack of personal fulfillment that she just couldn't bring herself to relax for moments of intimacy, alone or with her partner.

I knew that she needed a way out. Upon our first visit together, I suggested to her that the issues in her tissues correlated with the issues in her life. The ideas we have within and the dreams we hold are real; they need our attention and, above all, an outlet for expression. The cysts that were developing around her ovaries represented unfinished business. Erica needed to write again, and I told her so. When we start cultivating something, then put it on hold and never allow it to fully develop, we see the physical manifestation of that lodged inside our tissues, particularly the reproductive tissues, since this is the area where growth takes shape in the body in spirit, ideation, and flesh. The cysts were dreams unrealized. In Erica's case, the writing projects—the book project she had shelved, her journals that had gotten tossed into storage, never to see the light of day—were like small buds in a garden, ready to surface but suddenly strangled by weeds, unwatered and denied sunlight.

I was convinced that Erica needed to exit the torturing comfort of the real-estate workforce to instead explore her passion and dive into her purpose. I was convinced that her healing would stem from the process of letting go, of softening, of allowance. Rather than forcing deals in her favor and *making shit happen*, she could live a life where she did what she wanted and let things start to happen through her. I was convinced that this surrender would also grant Erica a sense of grounding and control that she sought in her life. I supported her for a nine-month transition out of her real-estate career and into writing. She got better sleep at night, her moods shifted, she started to have less painful periods and actually invite intimacy, her hormones slowly fell back into balance, her stress levels reduced dramatically, and her cysts shrank in diameter.

Erica ultimately took steps toward wombifesting her dreams. She had faith in my process for her and took refuge in slowing down and cultivating from within. She found her solace in the creative process of writing. When she finally surrendered herself to "less doing and more being," she became more aligned with her internal rhythms, allowing everything to fall into place.

There is a very primal desire in each of us to create something, to leave a mark on the world. I believe we accomplish this through our projects, our passions, and, many times, even our pleasures. But what happens if you shut off that faucet of creativity? Where does all the creative energy get stored? You can have it all; you just can't do it all at once. So, what will you give up so you can have the life you dream of? How will you open up? What part of you needs to be more pliant?

I believe it starts with slowing down a tad and looking within, developing the practices on the yoga mat and in your personal life, that will sustain you on this journey of personal growth and ultimate glow power. This is what wombifestation is all about—gestating from within, being your own source of light and being comfortable with slowing down and stillness.

The Gift of Slowing Down

We are living the fast life instead of the good life. We are rushing through life instead of relishing life. Our roadrunner, accelerated culture is taking over. Our time in the Western world is linear, and it is completely running us into the ground. Accelerated living does come at a cost. When we have to schedule sex and compromise sleep because time is evading us, it's time to reevaluate what's truly important. Believe it or not, the quality of your work improves the less you work and the more fun you have. And it's not just adults who are hurried and harried; even the children in our culture are overworked. Instead, we need to adopt a "less is more" mentality.

Slower is almost always better. You can't rush a cake that needs to bake! Everything worth cultivating takes time, and we should embrace the slowness. Slowness is a taboo in our culture, a concept associated with laziness and lethargy and a lack of intelligence or complexity. But we would be wise to slow down in order to perform better, eat better, and love better. Hurry up and slow down. To slow down is to be dialed into awareness, intention, and introspection.

Awareness. Many of us shuffle through our days, unaware of the distractions around us. From the first blare of the alarm clock thrusting us into an already accelerated day to listening to the news in a taxicab while texting, we are constantly wired to some sort of stimulus, whether we realize it or not.

Begin to practice slowing down and stillness by simply observing. See how long you can ride the subway without texting or playing a video game, or see how long you can drive in silence without the radio or talking on the phone. Can you sit and watch a program without changing the station? Can you forgo watching TV at all? Can you cook a meal without distraction or eat without checking your email? Build in buffering boundaries for awareness, perhaps muting commercials when watching TV, working out without your headphones, reading a book instead of surfing the Net. When you are out in public, take the lead and make eye contact with others, smile, and lift your head up from your phone for a change.

Intentionality. Undivided attention is a gift. The next time you're with a friend, offer him or her all your attention. Turn your phone off, log off of Instagram, and don't tweet or answer texts. The tether of social media is quite alluring and addicting, but there are studies that show that our obsession with social media and immediacy of communication has a profound impact on our mood. Allow the experience you are having to be worthy of your full attention and presence. Forget about your Facebook status and check the status within. Focus on preserving the quality of relationships you have at hand. Don't just give attention based on popularity, likes, hearts, or comments in the virtual world. Instead, give your attention based on genuine caring and being in the moment. Actively challenge the feelings that come up from not knowing what others are up to by not constantly checking in on others' social-media feeds. The truth is that social media allows us to curate what we present, but it's not an offering of complete transparency. People show what they want us to see. Whatever that is, it certainly isn't worth the distraction from what you have going on in the moment.

Introspection. Being alone is a terrifying idea for so many women I've come in contact with. Learning to spend time with yourself and carving out time to be alone is an important part of cultivating your glow power. The more you are comfortable with yourself—your power, your purpose—the stronger your connection to your GPS. Deep breathing, journaling, meditation, running, silence—these solo activities put us in touch with our dreams and amplify our feelings. Creativity is often sparked when self-awareness is heightened. When we allow ourselves to detach from the hustle of our modern lives, to be still and engage with what's going on inside, then we find the inspiration, motivation, and strong sense of self-worth necessary for dialing up our glow power. You might use introspective time to ignite your ritual practice—cleanse with a bath or thorough sage smudging, set an intention, meditate, visualize or feel the elements you are igniting, and be still within. Introspection allows us to keep the flame within ablaze.

The Lunar Cycle and Your Rhythms

My work is all about awakening the rhythmic cycles of the divine feminine within. We've just covered wombifestation and explored slowing down and expanding our creative power. We've tuned in to our GPS to deepen self-discovery. Now it's time we acknowledge and learn from the universe's other feminine force that influences us—the moon and its phases.

The moon—*la luna, la lune*. As the nearest natural satellite to Earth, appearing bigger than any star in our sky apart from the sun, the moon is a strong celestial force. Its mystical energy continuously affects our modern lives. The moon governs the waters, and its gravitational pull causes the tides. And since the human body, much like the Earth, is made up of roughly 70 percent water, we too are affected by the moon.

Women, more so than men, are said to feel this connection more aptly. A woman's menstrual cycle, on average running 28 days, mirrors the moon's approximate 29-day orbit around the earth. The word *menstruation* is etymologically related to the word "moon," and *menses* is derived from the Latin word *mensis*, which means "month," and is related to *mene*, which means "moon" in Greek. In ancient times, women were thought to have their menstrual cycles all at the same time, in alignment with each other and with the moon's phases. Women often spent time together in sacred spaces during their cycles. The idea that menstruation is or ought to be in harmony with wider cosmic rhythms is one of the most tenacious ideas central to the myths and rituals of traditional communities across the globe. The essence of the moon is inextricably aligned with the feminine. Have you ever experienced the feeling of being more alive, excitable, or aroused during a full moon? Each moon phase emanates a different type of energy, which can be harnessed and applied to your life. We can increase well-being, productivity, and glow power by closely charting the lunar cycles.

New Moon

The new moon is her darkest phase, where she is not visible. The pull of the moon during this phase invites you to look at your darkness, summon your inner light, face your fears, mourn your losses, and examine your mistakes. This moon provides us with hope for new beginnings. It's a great time for formulating creative endeavors and setting intentions for career advancement. You can chart the course for a new project. Reevaluate your goals, plans, and dreams. It's about planting seeds of optimism. The new moon invites us to examine deep-rooted beliefs and unearth them to move forward. It's a great time to set intentions that honor and elevate your spiritual practice. Prayer, divination work, visual art, and dream interpretation are all beneficial self-care practices that may help ease fatigue. There is a lot of mystery around the darkness of a new moon. It's aligned with birth and the beginning of our feminine phases. It's a gateway from the old to the new and a time to fully release what's past and plant seeds for what's to come. It's a time for introspection.

Feeling: You are likely to be most introverted and self-absorbed during this time. This is when energy is the most subdued. You are likely to feel more emotional and sensitive; you may feel mentally checked out and not focused on completing tasks.

Doing: Dream more, do less! This is the time to rest! Give yourself the permission to do creative things—like vision-boarding, for example—that nurture you, allowing you to set intentions and goals. Gather with supportive and like-minded women. Reconcile with the past. Meditate and pray. Do not launch anything new—but you can announce what's to come. Invite new energy into your life. Just be in this energy of clarity and dreaming. Take care of you.

Being: Be still and contemplative.

Waxing Crescent Moon, Waxing Half-Moon, Waxing Gibbous Moon

The waxing moon phase means increasing energy, alongside building and growing. This phase is aligned with the maiden archetype and aids the accomplishments of new undertakings. This is the time when you walk through that open door of opportunity. Seeds are germinating underground and getting ready to peek through the damp, dark dirt you planted during the new moon. Projects build momentum; if you've been taking action, now is the time you begin to see the rudiments of results. This is a great time to start a new health regimen, hone work habits, and socialize with a supportive group of friends or network. Cultivate budding new relationships, especially romantic ones. You might update your resume or redesign your website to attract new work opportunities. It's also a time of intense attraction, both positive and negative. Pay close attention to your thoughts—are they positive? What's pulling your attention? If it's positive, that is what you will attract. Are your actions grounded in love? These are the seeds you are sowing that will bloom upon the Full Moon. This process should be conscious. Everything happening in your life is a result of what you have put there and what you have nurtured and allowed to flourish in your life. This is a time to put new intentions into action, to encourage healthy, sustainable patterns. Energy turns into form during this phase. The momentum of the waxing moon will help you put your new rituals into practice.

Feeling: You feel more engaged, with a deep need to prepare and set things in order. Your energy is rising, and you feel more capable of getting more done.

Doing: Put structure and plans into motion, align your actions with goals and intentions set during the new moon. Update services, schedule meetings, communicate new ideas, write down thoughts for new projects, and delegate tasks. Essentially, plant more seeds and water the soil.

Being: Now is the time to be open and receptive.

Full Moon

The Full Moon is the phase most are familiar with, when she's biggest and brightest in the sky. You're pregnant, so to speak, with all that energy and light. You're supported by the light. This moon phase is aligned with our fertile mother and nurturer energy. Intentions you planted at the New Moon have come to fruition. All that light in the sky shines on Earth, and what was hidden is revealed. People tend to go a little bit crazy at the full moon: have you ever heard of *luna*tics? It's a highly electrifying time packed with energy and a good time to go on dates, flirt, and be outwardly expressive. This is a great time to make presentations at work, ask for a raise, or interview for a new position. Acknowledge your accomplishments. This is harvest time. Pull the energy of the full moon to help bring your desires wombifest. Be mindful to ground that energy and use it for the highest good. The full moon is a reminder of who you are at the fullest and who you are becoming. It's a time of prophecy and divination, for you can see most clearly under the light of the full moon.

Feeling: You are feeling creative, inspired, expansive, nurturing, and productive. This is the peak energy of the cycle. You are radiant, most confident, and adventurous during this phase. If your cycle is aligned with the moon, then this is your period of ovulation.

Doing: Work and play hard, have fun, create and launch new programs, write new blog posts, journal, and complete the tasks you dreamed about during the new-moon phase. This is a great time for pitch meetings and presentations and to complete work already begun. Use the upward-and-outward energy that you are getting from the moon to help you move forward. Harvest what you've planted.

Being: Be active and outgoing.

Waning Gibbous Moon, Waning Half-Moon, Waning Crescent Moon

This is the moon phase associated with the Crone, or with wise, elderly-woman energy. The energy from the full moon starts to die down while journeying back toward becoming the new moon. It's a meditative time when you are supported to release patterns, addictions, thoughts, behaviors, and relationships—all the things that don't serve you. It's the "let go" moon phase or the "take no shit" phase. This moon calls for intuitive reflection and cutting ties. This is a great time to cleanse, as our bodies are most susceptible to detoxification during this phase. What the phases of the moon reveal to us is that there is wisdom hidden in the vacuum of the darkness. We can't always be full and light; there is a time for the shadow to reign. We must have time to go into the dark and be born anew. We empty out to be full again. We fall apart to come back together again; we come together again to fall apart. She is full of endless mystery and magic, dark and light, just like the magical mystery that you are, divine woman.

Feeling: You have a strong desire to clear. Energy levels recede as you transition from the full-moon peak to the new-moon low, with a desire to tie up loose ends and fix things that aren't working.

Doing: Meditate and recalibrate. Wrap up things and complete tasks, especially anything that has been weighing on you. Invoice clients, clear your desk and closets, banish any clutter, and take care of any to-dos that will prevent you from feeling restful and peaceful during the coming new-moon phase. Weed and till the soil.

Being: You feel mysterious and withdrawn.

Black Moon (Dark Moon)

This quiet period is just two to three days before the new moon, when the last slivers of the waning moon disappear. The dark moon prompts us to examine what isn't working and to release, as well as explore, emerging seed goals and desires that we may want to plant and initiate during the new moon. Integrating our darkness is a key component of our transformation. It's in the power of this phase that we can unload, lean deeply into the unknown, and begin again. Shed the patterns, people, and behaviors that create discord in your life and use the powerful energy of the black moon to help you. Call on your ancestors or guides to protect you during this period of release. Uncomfortable truths are difficult to avoid, so use this energy to wrap up whatever has run its course.

Feeling: You may feel emotional and highly sensitive with an urge to clear up areas of your life that have been calling for your attention.

Doing: Access what you need to let go and write a list and game plan. Releasing blame, shame, and guilt and practicing forgiveness are recommended during this time. Drink herbal tea like nettle and yarrow infusions. Get good rest and go to bed earlier than usual. You might burn mugwort, which supports clarity in dreaming. Record your dreams and journal. This is a good time to retreat and take a fast from your phone and other electronic devices.

Being: Be clear and complete.

New- and Full-Moon Rituals

As new moons represent fresh starts and new beginnings, full moons mark wombifestation and moments of completion. Setting intentions and grounding yourself in rituals during these potent periods can help you harness your glow power.

Create a sacred space. Find a quiet place to sit. Place crystals, flowers, or other special objects around you or at your altar. Light candles.

Clear your energy. Light a smudge stick to clear the air. Imagine standing under a cascading waterfall and allow all negative or blocking forces to be washed away.

Set your intentions. Write down what you are cultivating for the new moon or celebrating or releasing on the full moon.

Make space for mindfulness. Sit in silence or with sound, where you can feel the supercharged new moon or be under the light of the full moon. Perhaps recite a mantra or affirmation, sing a song, or read poetry.

Play music and move. Get your body moving while playing some grounding and sensual music. Try primal movement on your hands and knees; close your eyes and do hip swivels. Make shapes that mimic nature. Be free with your body.

Give thanks. Gratitude is one of the most powerful tools in our arsenal. When we give thanks for each of the lessons, teachers, challenges, and triumphs we have encountered, we create space for more goodness.

Use your intuition to guide you to create a constellation of meaningful rituals for your own life.

RITUAL
HOSTING A MOON GATHERING

Calling all sisters! Share your intention in the safety of a circle of women. Attend or host your own new or full-moon circle. This is a ritually charged gathering that allows you to be in support of other women and explore the ever-changing currents of womanhood and the cyclical nature of the moon. Whether you are hosting a new or full-moon gathering, consider the following to create a soulful and grounding experience for all:

Set the mood. Consider the theme for your gathering. Is it the full or new moon? What season are you in? In what setting or space will you be hosting the event? What colors, symbols, or decor feel appropriate for this particular moon gathering? Will you serve food? What will be on the menu? Will there be a dress code? Who will you invite? This is the fun part of planning your moon gathering.

Create an altar. Build an altar based on the theme of the gathering and ask guests to bring a sacred or symbolic object to place at the altar. Choice objects might include flowers, seashells, feathers, rocks, or crystals surrounded by candles.

Create safe spaces for vulnerability. Sharing a meal at the beginning of the circle is a great way to gather people and encourage them to be open. Nurture your guests through grounding arts and crafts that support the theme and allow ample time for them to settle in and get comfortable.

Cleanse. Using sage, *palo santo*, or any incense or resin of choice, smudge each guest before they enter the circle. You can silently speak a blessing upon each person as you smudge them.

Consider your playlist. Music has an effect on our emotions. And both the new and full moons have a way of bringing our emotions to the surface. Put a playlist together that evokes the elements of nature—earth, air, fire, water, and ether—to take your guests on a journey.

Create a cozy circle. Place pillows or cushions and blankets on the ground in the shape of a circle. Have everyone place their object of significance in the center of the altar.

Open the circle. The sense of safety and belonging that guests feel will depend upon who is facilitating the circle. The facilitator will hold space for the group. The circle can be initiated with a prayer, poetry, or a talk exploring the theme of the gathering. Have guests explore the theme through a writing or sharing.

Moonifest and release. Allow everyone the opportunity to either speak aloud or draft their intentions and what they are cultivating and making moonifest. Then have them share something they are ready to release from their lives.

Revel. Relax, dance, imbibe, and celebrate the magic of the moment and revel in the energy that was cultivated in this sacred gathering.

Close the circle. Give each guest a small token to take home from the gathering that embodies the theme. Close with a reflection, meditation, or prayer summoning the communal support of each other.

The Pull from Within

We've learned about the feminine energy of the moon and how we can best align our process—the steps we take toward achieving our purpose—with the moon's phases. Let's turn our attention inward. We embody feminine forces of our own. We'll further explore our sacred spaces—including gaining an understanding of how our own menstrual cycles affect the work we do in the same way the lunar cycle does—and that the exploration begins with a study of our own sacred anatomy. The word ritual comes from *rtu*, Sanskrit for "menses." Some of the earliest rituals were connected to the menstrual cycle. The blood from the womb was believed to be magical and sacred. How familiar are you with your innermost parts? Most of what we have been taught about our bodies has come from textbooks and television, advertisements, doctors and experts, hearsay from friends, and columns in magazines. We're taught that our bodies are flawed, dirty, and wild and need to be controlled. Let's flip that notion and explore the magic of our own internal rhythms and how reclaiming this connection can solidify our intentions, ground our seed goals, boost our confidence, and amplify our glow power.

Your Sacred Anatomy

Lily, papaya, Padma, rose, magnolia flower, box, cave, secret garden, cookie, dark gate, black hole, heavenly gate, trap, pussy, sacred passageway . . . so many words to describe your inner sanctum, the vagina. The word *vagina* originates from Latin, meaning "sheath," particularly to a man's "sword." The now-controversial word *cunt* is derived from the name of the venerated Greek goddess of fertility Kunthus and also of Kunti, an Indian goddess of nature and earth. Cultures throughout the world have been using language to show reverence for the female body since the beginning of time, but we've also been using language rooted in denouncing the female body for centuries.

It's important to know what the words you are using mean, where they come from, and what they symbolize. Are you using language that perpetuates a legacy of misogyny, or are you using language to reframe and reclaim your sacred body parts? In Sanskrit, *yoni*—the downward-pointing triangle—symbolizes the womb, and each letter of the word has an esoteric meaning that celebrates the magic and mystery of the womb. There is also the pointed oval, which symbolizes the vulva. The yoni was recognized as the seat of feminine sexual power. Tantric practitioners believed this power was the source of *all* creative action. The female orgasm was regarded as the most energizing force of the universe. The female center was not seen as passive, but a wild and animated force.

Learning about our bodies and the place from which all of us come—the origin and source of all life, the divine feminine—is key.

We learn about our bodies through our partners, many of whom have no better understanding of our complex systems than we do because we haven't learned ourselves. On the whole, we don't get wisdom passed down from our elders about our bodies. When you visit your gynecologist, there are posters of the reproductive system on the walls, showing the uterus, fallopian tubes, and the vaginal passageway and vulva, but there's nothing about the arousal system or erectile network. We learn nothing about anatomic variability and how that is reflected in our vulvas. Why is this information kept tucked away?

Casper Bartholin, Gabriele Falloppio, and Ernst Gräfenberg—what do all these names have in common? You have likely never heard of any of these people, yet you have body parts named after each of these *men*. Our sacred female anatomy has been colonized and named after men who don't even have our body parts. The sacred female anatomy is complex, and the scope is far beyond what I will touch on here, but I would be remiss if I didn't uncover the sacred matrix that is your wombiverse. Let's explore the sunshine that lies between your thighs.

Your Wombiverse

Pubis—The triangle containing scent glands, covering the mons veneris and labia majora. Sometimes covered in hair, unless you wax or shave.

Mons veneris—The "mount of Venus," or mons pubis, is a cushion of fatty tissue that protects the pubic bones and splits to become the labia majora. This small bump of flesh on the pubic bone is the latest body part that women now hate. There's even a cosmetic procedure to "fix" it known as *monsplasty* (or "a pubic") to reduce and tighten the mons pubis.

Labia majora—The large outer lips of the vagina extending from the mons veneris to the perineum, containing oil-secreting scent glands and sweat glands. The labia majora engorges during arousal.

Labia minora—The small inner lips colored in various shades of pink or brown, containing scent glands and sweat glands. They can swell up to three times normal size during sexual arousal and join to form the clitoral hood. The labia minora lead to the vaginal opening.

Clitoral hood—A small mobile foreskin that covers the shaft of the clitoris. It forms a protective hood over the clitoral crown.

Clitoral crown—The clitoral crown is the visible part of what many think is the entire clitoris, but it's just the tip of the iceberg. It is our most sensitive erogenous zone and generally considered the primary source of female sexual pleasure. The clitoris is a complex structure, and its size and sensitivity can vary. During arousal, the crown projects itself far outside the clitoral hood. The crown of the clitoris is roughly the size and shape of a pea and is estimated to have more than 8,000 sensory nerve endings. It's designed for pleasure.

Clitoral legs—Until psychologist-anatomist-sexologist Josephine Lowndes Sevely came along, it was believed that only women have clitorises. Well, now we know that men have them, too. Sevely theorized that the male *corpora cavernosa*, a pair of sponge-like regions of erectile tissue that sustain the blood in the penis during penile erection, are the true counterpart of the clitoris. The clitoris consists of a shaft and legs shaped like a wishbone, and is a large structure of erectile tissue. Each leg runs downward around the vestibular bulbs and along the sides of the labia majora. The clitoral legs become enlarged and tremble involuntarily when touched during high-level arousal and orgasm.

Vestibular bulbs (Bartholin's glands)—These glands are located between the vaginal wall and the labia minora. They secrete a protein compound through the vestibular ducts and into the vestibule. They lubricate the vaginal opening and stimulate sexual scent. They are connected to the fertility cycle, the scent glands, and pheromone attraction. When aroused, these glands engorge, making for more cushioned walls within the vagina for intercourse.

Vaginal glans—A highly sensitive zone located below the clitoral crown and above the vaginal opening. It is sensitive and flexible, and during intercourse, it moves in and out of the vagina, creating a pleasurable sensation for the woman.

Vestibule—Also called the vulva, this is the outer part of the vagina surrounded by the labia minora and containing openings to the urethra, vagina, and the ducts from the vestibular bulbs. The Chinese refer to this portal of the body as "the heavenly court."

Vagina—An expansive, muscular space connecting the opening or vestibule to the cervix. It is the sacred passageway by which many of us traveled to be born. Highly lubricated by its mucous membranes, it is the pathway that monthly menses travels and the route sperm cells take on their way to the egg.

Perineum—The flesh located between the vaginal opening and the anus. It's often considered a no-man's-land, but it's a highly sensitive region and loaded with erectile tissue. The Chinese consider the ovaries and the perineum the seat of Yin energy (a downward-pointing triangle connects these parts). Far too often, the perineum is cut to enlarge the vaginal space to accommodate the head of a baby at birth. This tissue is very sensitive and should remain intact.

Perineal sponge—Sensitive erectile tissue beneath the perineum that engorges during arousal, creating more cushion at the base of the vagina in preparation for intercourse.

Urethra—In both women and men, the urethra transports urine from the bladder toward its opening. It's surrounded by the urethral sponge.

Urethral sponge—Consisting of glands, blood vessels, flesh, and paraurethral glands and ducts, its stimulation and arousal can be instrumental in reaching orgasm and releasing female orgasmic fluids. The engorgement of the urethral sponge creates what's known as the G-spot, a sensitive area named after Ernst Gräfenberg. To be clear, the G-spot is not a place; it's a state of arousal. If the urethral sponge is not engorged and you simply have sex without being fully aroused, you won't feel the pleasure associated with this erotogenic pressure point.

Prostatic glands—It was once believed that only men had prostate glands. Now we know there are prostatic glands in women connected by a large number of ducts to the urethra, transporting glandular fluids and elements that make female ejaculate.

Cervical os—The mouth of the uterus, this is the gateway from the vagina into the uterus. It cannot be penetrated through intercourse. After childbirth, it seals tightly shut once again.

Cervix—The neck of the uterus, it projects forward into the vagina. It dilates open to 10 centimeters, releasing an infant into the vagina for delivery. The os and the cervix are the mouth and throat of the reproductive system and are hard-wired to our actual mouth and throat. When we relax the mouth and throat, we relax the pelvic floor and cervix.

Uterus—The uterus, the womb, includes the cervical os and the cervix and is a hollow muscle the size of an avocado. It shifts in dimension and orientation based on arousal. The inner lining of the uterus, known as the endometrium, undergoes several changes throughout the moon cycle. The uterus expands up to 500 times its normal size to accommodate a growing baby and begins contracting immediately after birth, resuming its normal size within weeks postpartum. Connected to the round ligaments, the uterus tilts rhythmically at orgasm. Ninety percent of all hysterectomies, in which the uterus is removed, are for non-cancerous reasons—because of fibroids, endometriosis, and uterine prolapse. Women are routinely told that they do not need their uteri, that the uterus is only for growing babies. On the contrary, the uterus is a power player in fertility and arousal.

Fallopian tubes—These egg-transporting tubes connect the ovaries to the upper end of the uterus and guide the eggs toward it. They are named after the Italian anatomist Gabriele Falloppio.

Ovaries—The ovaries are part of the endocrine system and not only produce eggs but also an array of sex hormones including estrogen, estradiol, and progesterone. Ovarian activity is governed synergistically by the pituitary hormones FSH (follicle-stimulating hormone), LH (luteinizing hormone), and PRL (prolactin). During ovulation, an egg is selected to float out of the ovaries and into one of the fallopian tubes for fertilization.

Pelvic floor—A complex system of muscles providing support for the pelvic organs, including the bladder and uterus. To avoid incontinence and to have better sex, women are taught to tone these muscles through Kegel exercises. Pelvic pumping increases circulation, stimulates nerves, increases arousal, and turns on the brain.

This system is highly sensitive, integrative, and complex. It is a world to uncover and explore by yourself first and with your partner. Your feminine topography is unique and an interconnected, whole system designed for pleasure, bliss, birth, and bonding. You don't have to experience all these pathways, but your body is capable and hardwired for each. Learn and love your body and all of your intricate parts.

Your Sacred Cycle

The menstrual cycle is governed by interactions between the hypothalamus gland, which is located deep within the brain; the pituitary gland, located at the base of the brain; and the ovaries. This trifecta works together to form a loop of coordinated hormonal messages upon which the health and stability of your cycle depends. The accompanying hormonal changes influence the way we feel. Some women feel a release of tension but an overwhelming feeling of fatigue and lack of focus.

I remember when I used to be merely annoyed at the thought of my cycle approaching. I would roll my eyes at the inconvenience. I had a relatively smooth and pain-free cycle throughout my teens and into college. It wasn't until I entered my sophomore year of college that I experienced my first bout of menstrual cramps. I was asleep and felt these sharp pains in my lower abdomen. I tossed and turned throughout the early morning until I was thrust into wakefulness. What could this be? I started praying, as if this was some indication that my life was coming to an end. I called my mother in a panic. "Mom, I think I'm dying. I am in so much pain." My mother explained to me that the sensations were in fact menstrual cramps and that most women feel them and that I was lucky to have only begun getting cramps then. *Wait, you call this lucky?* I thought.

Well, it was a totally different ball game now that I had cramps. I once had to leave a grocery store in the middle of my weekly shopping trip, doubled over in pain. I didn't like the fact that I was subject to the "whims" of my body. But I came to learn that proper nutrition and self-care, acupuncture, and the elimination of sweets leading up to the cycle and afterward could eliminate my cramps, PMS, and leave me feeling restored.

Your body speaks the truth; it does not lie. It asks for what it wants, and, if you are compliant, your body will continue to function at peak levels, supporting you and your mission. If you deny your body adequate rest, fortifying foods, energizing and restorative movement, pleasure, and good company, your hormones will hijack your mood, your energy levels, and your metabolism, and your inner witch will come home to roost. Our bleeding is a portal to deepening our intuition and solidifying the self-care continuum. The menstrual cycle is a sacred event that we are blessed to undergo. Yes, blessed! Each cycle promises a potential new life, and when it passes, that life force is lost and the body mourns it. We are more emotionally and energetically sensitive during this period. Our senses are heightened, and, as with the changing moon phases, our fluctuating hormones lead to shifts in the nature of our interactions and our consciousness. Not every woman bleeds and not everyone who bleeds is a woman. Your intrinsic worth has nothing to do with your ability to bleed or give birth.

There is a wealth of information published on the many taboos associated with menstruation and the immense power attributed to it by world cultures. Menstrual fluid was believed to have adverse effects on humans, animals, and nature. Menstruating women were often separated from their tribes and families out of fear. Other ancient cultures believed that menstrual fluid was infused with unique powers. They held menstruating women in high regard.

Among the Incas, Mama Kilya, the moon goddess, was worshipped as the ruler of the menstrual cycle. The alchemists recognized the potent energy of menstrual blood. Ancient Egyptians wore amulets of red stone that represented the powers of the menstrual blood of their most exalted goddess, Isis. In ancient Persia, in pre-patriarchal times, the goddess Jaki was thought to be responsible for menstruation. Native American menstrual rites often included visits to menstrual huts. During the heaviest four days of their periods, women would leave their homes and go to this separate menstrual lodge to commune with other women. They were not allowed to prepare meals or do household work; they focused on visioning and rest. Women of many cultures would spread their menses in fields to make them fertile. Now we know that menses is full of stem cells and is actually a great fertilizer. Our blood is life.

Menstruation and the Triple Goddess

I want to introduce you now to your cycle through the lens of the Triple Goddess, the trinity corresponding to the three visible phases of the moon and mirroring the three major phases in the life of a woman: prepubescent girl or maiden (waxing crescent moon), menstruating fertile woman or mother (full moon), and postmenopausal wise crone or sage (waning crescent moon). There is a sacred feminine presence in the form of a Trifecta that can be found across all cultures. The Celtic/Welsh goddesses Blodeuwedd (goddess of beauty, spring, and flowers), Arianrhod (goddess of fertility, rebirth, and destiny), and Cerridwen (goddess of knowledge and light) are part of the Druan Gwen, or Triple Goddess. The West African tradition of Ifa' has Oshun (goddess of sweetness and fertility), Yemanja, (goddess of fortune and the mother), and Yansá (goddess of tempests and thunder). We find manifestations of these goddesses in Haitian, Afro-Cuban, and Brazilian cultures. And in the Indian Hindu tradition, where we'll set our focus, we see the three goddesses who are all facets of Shakti—the female principle, the Yin. Those goddesses are: Durga (destruction/clearance), Saraswati (education/ sustenance/ flow), and Lakshmi (creation/abundance/prosperity). The phases of the triple goddess are not fixed on our chronological age but rather correspond to where we are in our lives. For instance, you could be moving through a wise-crone phase and be in your 30s or celebrating a maiden aspect in your 70s. Each of these goddesses represents a facet of your sacred cycle. Let's break them down.

Durga and the shedding phase. Goddess Durga is the dynamic mother of the Universe and is believed to be the power behind the work of the creation, preservation, and destruction of the world. Durga is associated with the dark underbelly of the moon. She is the goddess of destruction and is associated with the breakdown of uterine lining and menstrual flow. The irritability associated with PMS is aligned with her energy. Durga clears all stagnant energies as well. This first phase of the cycle, which lasts an average of five to seven days, begins with the first day of our menstrual flow and is an opportunity for us to clear out and let go. Like a forest fire that is set ablaze, the energy of Durga can often clear things we might not have the ability to clear out on our own.

Glow protocol: During this phase of your cycle, allow yourself to rest, and refrain from doing any strenuous physical activity. Instead, take a leisurely walk and get fresh air. Feed yourself blood-building, robust foods, including green juice, beets, squashes, and avocado, and adequate protein through smoothies and light snacks throughout the day. Sip on infused ginger tea to help ease any cramps. Make an effort to be in bed before 10 P.M., and if you have any major commitments, play hooky!

Power themes: Release and Let Go.

Yoga poses: To relieve menstrual cramps and tension in the lower back and to rest the brain—triangle pose (*utthita trikonasana*), half-moon pose (*ardha chandrasana*), forward fold (*uttanasana*), and child's pose (*adho mukha virasana*).

Essential-oil blend: Clary sage, lavender, bergamot, Roman chamomile, cedarwood, ylang-ylang, geranium, fennel, carrot seed. Placed over the abdomen, this blend helps release stress and tension and is a powerful emotional stabilizer during menstruation and perimenopause.

Ritual: Banish stagnant energy and write down the negative things that you would like to eliminate. Then burn that piece of paper. Do an at-home spa treatment, scrub and exfoliate, and then moisturize. Have a cup of herbal tea to soothe and relax.

Mantra: *I release and let go of what no longer fulfills me.*

Saraswati and the renewal phase. The goddess Saraswati is aligned with cultivation, the arts, and inspiration. The Sanskrit word *sara* means "essence," and *swa* means "self." She represents the free flow of wisdom and consciousness. It is believed that goddess Saraswati endows human beings with the powers of speech, wisdom, and learning. She has four hands representing the four aspects of human personality in learning: mind, intellect, alertness, and ego. She is represented with sacred scriptures in one hand and a lotus—the symbol of true knowledge—in a second. With her remaining two hands, she plays the music of love and life on a string instrument called the *veena*. She is often depicted dressed in white, the color of purity. She is a portal of renewal, beauty, and restored energy post menses. Once you are done bleeding, you enter the Saraswati phase, when you suddenly regain your cognitive energy, you want to get back into the gym, your memory is sharper, your state of mind is more outgoing and expressive, and you feel like a new person. Because you are! This restoration period lasts about seven days and starts the day your period ends and moves you into ovulation.

Glow protocol: During this second phase of your cycle, begin incorporating more physically challenging activities. You can get back to the treadmill, your power-yoga sequences, CrossFit, and whatever else you love during this phase. A jump-rope or trampoline session to music will reflect the pep in your step that you may be experiencing from entering the Saraswati phase. Read a good book, play chess, watch a new mystery series, and engage your intellect. Eat heartier meals containing healthy fats like avocado, walnuts, quinoa, black beans, and almonds. One of my favorite recipes for rosemary almonds comes from Alicia Keys. It's one of my go-to glow foods to carry while in the renewal phase. It's made with peeled almonds, rosemary, olive oil, and sea salt. Have a smoothie containing low-glycemic berries like blueberries, along with hempseed oil and *maca* powder (an adaptogen that works on the reproductive system). Goji-berry tea helps to restore the body after menses and offers an array of amino acids. Simply place 2 tsp of dried goji berries into a cup of boiling water. Allow them to soak and release their power into the water, then drink.

Power themes: Uplift and Restore

Yoga poses: To boost blood circulation, balance the hormones and increase energy—downward-facing dog (*adho mukha svanasana*), wide-leg straddle stretch (*prasarita paddottanasana*), child's pose (*adho mukha virasana*), and leg drain (*viparita karani*).

Essential-oil blend: Wild orange, lemon, grapefruit, mandarin, bergamot, and tangerine. This blend placed over the solar plexus encourages grounding, self-confidence, and invigoration.

Ritual: Embrace the energy of renewal and burn a candle. Journal on gratitude with a hot cup of tea.

Mantra: *I am restored in mind, spirit, and flesh.*

Lakshmi and the fertile phase. The name *Lakshmi* is derived from the Sanskrit word *laksya*, meaning "aim" or "goal," and she is the goddess of wealth and prosperity both material and spiritual. Lakshmi is depicted as a beautiful woman with a golden complexion and four hands, sitting or standing on a full-bloomed lotus and holding a lotus bud, which stands for beauty, purity, and fertility. Her four hands represent the four ends of human life: *dharma*, or righteousness; *kama*, or desires; *artha*, or wealth; and *moksha*, or liberation from the cycle of birth and death. Lakshmi holds the promise of material fulfillment and embodies the fertile nature of the earth itself. In this third ovulatory phase of your cycle, you can stay out much later, as you have the energy and desire—flirt if you're single, dress up and enjoy yourself. In addition to the recharged energy levels, you will also enjoy a libido boost and notice you are more radiant—your complexion may be clearer and cheeks flushed, giving you a natural glow. The sensuality of the goddess is part of her potency. Ovulation can occur on any one day between 11 and 21 on a 28-day cycle.

Glow protocol: During this phase of your cycle, you're physically more attractive in appearance than any other time—this is a scientific fact. You have an urge to be more outgoing and more sensual as your fertility window heightens your sensitivity. Take a sensual dance class like Pole or S-Factor, salsa, belly dancing, or tango. In your ancestral wiring, there are attunement processes that are underway when you start dancing, when you are in pulsation. Go to the ocean and walk along the beach. If you aren't near a body of water, take a warm salt bath with rose petals. Sing, whether in the shower alone or with an audience at karaoke. When you sing, hum, or chant, you invoke an aspect and vibration of the goddess, so we can see her full expression. Recommended foods for this period include sweet potatoes, cacao, *maca*-root powder, coconut oil, dates, and leafy greens.

Power themes: Create and Flow

Yoga poses: To boost blood circulation in the pelvis and increase energy—seated forward fold (*upavistha konasana*), extended angle (*utthita parsvakonasana*), downward-facing dog (*adho mukha svanasana*), and warrior II (*virabhadrasana* II).

Essential-oil blend: Patchouli, bergamot, sandalwood, rose, jasmine, cinnamon, vetiver, ylang-ylang. Placed on the abdomen and heart, this blend invites us to soften and connect with our sensuality.

Ritual: Celebrate the fertile and abundant energy of ovulation. Take an aromatic rose-petal bath by candlelight. Spray yourself with rose water. Wear red lipstick!

Mantra: *I am a creative matrix.*

MEDITATION
IGNITING THE PRESENCE OF THE TRIPLE GODDESS IN MY LIFE

Mother Spirit, in your greatness, please flank us with your eternal blessings.

Please help me clear all stagnant energies in my life that prevent the essence of Saraswati from settling in and bringing her gifts.

Please help me tune out so I can tune inward to the evanescent warmth of light and love sustained by the goddess.

Durga has cleared the path and removed so many things for me that I could not clear on my own, and now I emerge in a space ready to open to the full expression of Lakshmi and her abundance.

I open to that essence and rise up with grace to meet the Divine. In this moment, in this space, I ignite the goddess within and celebrate my own divinity.

Honoring Your Sacred Cycle

When we bleed, it is a sacred time, although it's often looked at as a curse. When a woman experiences PMS and a symptomatic cycle, it often means she is spreading herself too thin and not listening to her internal rhythms. Scheduling your life, as often as possible, so that you're not taxing yourself will keep you from senselessly depleting your energy during your cycle. When you feel tired, slow down. The body speaks in very clear terms about what it needs and desires from you. During your bleeding phase, it's time to dream more and sleep more. As you lose blood, you also lose minerals, and it's easy to feel depleted. Some women even become anemic. Carrying on as if nothing is happening will result in you pushing yourself too far, which in turn can result in moodiness, low blood sugar, and symptomatic headaches.

During your bleeding phase, just say no to everything. Even if you feel like you have the energy, allow yourself the opportunity to rest. A practice of setting boundaries, resting, dreaming, eating well, phone-fasting, and meditation will help you to get the most out of your bleeding phase and boost your glow power. Whenever possible, you should steer clear of making any major commitments that will create pressure or put you through unnecessary stress. For example, I will not take on any late client appointments or commit to evening events that will keep me out late at night during my period. I want to be finished with my workday by 3 P.M. I work from my desk at home the first two days of my period and temper this time with much-needed rest. I essentially mark a red line through the times when I bleed, and I request this of my clients as well. Reclaim that time to rest your body. What can you take a stand for? What will you stop doing during your bleeding phase? What can you let go of? This period is all about clearance.

White-Moon and Red-Moon Cycles

When women start tracking their periods with the lunar cycle, they fall into two categories: white-moon menstruation, which is bleeding with or near the new moon, and ovulating with the full moon, or red-moon menstruation, which is bleeding with or near the full moon and becoming fertile with the new moon. Your period will ebb and flow, attuning to both cycles during your lifetime for various reasons. Note what's going on in your life energetically as your body moves through these cycles. Notice the difference in your mood, your blood, menstrual symptoms, cravings, libido, and outlook when you bleed on the new moon versus the full moon. What is your body communicating through you?

If your body follows a white-moon cycle, you'll likely bleed during the waning or new moon. The earth is most fertile during the full moon. When you're ovulating, this cycle is inextricably connected to fertility and motherhood. You may experience a surge in your intuition during your period, and you will feel the urge to withdraw for self-care and self-renewal rituals.

If your body follows a red-moon cycle, you will likely bleed during the waxing or full moon and be most fertile during the new or waning moon. Full- and waxing-moon phase attributes include: being highly creative, outgoing, shining, and energetic. In ancient times, the red-moon cycle was associated with shamanic healers. Women who menstruate with the full moon are believed to harness their dark and creative energies and channel them outward, nourishing others and imparting wisdom from their own experience. Modern women with this cycle may have a focus on self-help, personal development, mentorship, and creativity.

You might find that as you increase awareness about your cycle, you have a preferred bleeding time. We'll explore how we can make modifications to our current lifestyle to align with the moon phase that best supports your needs, goals, and desires.

Syncing Your Cycle

There are ways to realign your cycle over time. Most moon rituals are performed during the new moon or full moon rather than during the waxing and waning phases, because the moon is at peak potency then. Those who love altars may find comfort in adorning theirs with red roses, rose quartz, moonstone, mother of pearl, or other symbols of fertility and immense feminine power. To the extent of your comfort level, incorporate the following practices to better sync your cycle and boost your glow power.

- **Sync your circadian rhythms.** Light modulates our bodies' natural rhythms. Our use of smartphones, computers, TVs, and the incessant exposure to artificial light impacts on our bodies. Sync your circadian rhythm by keeping your home flooded with sunlight light during daylight hours and dark during nighttime. Minimize your use of sunglasses, especially during ovulation, and keep lights dim or light candles at night.

- **Bask in a moon bath.** Moonlight also plays a role in our monthly rhythms. Research has shown that sleeping with a 100-watt light bulb on during the five to six days of the full moon—and sleeping in complete darkness for the rest of the month—regulates menstruation. Just being outside in natural moonlight is incredibly healthy physically and recharges us energetically: you may have the urge to go out dancing with friends during the full moon. You can place your crystals in the moonlight to charge them, too. Whether you spend time outside, attend a full-moon yoga class, or just open the blinds fully during her five days of luminosity, you will feel charged up.

- **Bring the outdoors indoors.** Get back to nature so your rhythms can get back on track. Open your windows and allow fresh air to flow along with the ambient sounds of nature or the city. Keep living houseplants in your bedroom and other spaces in your home to boost the presence of nature.

- **Practice self-care.** As I said before, it's essential that you reclaim your period as sacred time for yourself. The first three days of menstruation are usually the most intense physically as well as mentally and emotionally.

Take the space you need, remind your partner you need nurturing, and ask your friends to check on you. Order take-out, curl up on the couch, and catch up on your favorite sitcoms.

RITUAL
MAPPING YOUR SACRED CYCLE

Conscious calendaring is an act of self-care. Each time you enter the Durga phase of your cycle, when you begin to bleed, map it. I know so many women who have no idea when their periods are coming. So many of us are not at all attuned to the rhythmic cycles of our bodies. Do you know when to expect your period? Go to your calendar and consider the next three months. Take a good look at what your schedule looks like. You may not plan that far ahead, but for the purposes of this exercise, do so. Mark what date your period should start and end on the calendar.

For mapping, consider a special journal focused only on this exercise, or download a mobile app. And don't just take note of the days on which you bleed. Take the time daily to record your menstrual-cycle indicators: changes in mood, diet, sleep, exercise, attention span, dreams, and physical symptoms. The frequency and length of a period varies from woman to woman, and so will the associated indicators. For some women, tension, irritability, and cramping are the norm, while migraines, tender breasts, and moodiness may affect others. Simply record the indicators you experience, and after a few months, you will notice common trends and develop a deeper understanding of your body's testimony. You will emerge from this exercise empowered with womb wisdom. Mapping the changes that occur throughout the month gives insight about the timing of your period and also a keen awareness of your womb health. Everything we experience during the entire cycle provides us with a testimony about our body, mind, and spirit, so actively listen and feel your way through.

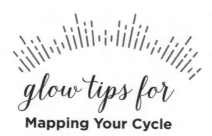

glow tips for
Mapping Your Cycle

Get to know your cervical fluid. Your cervical fluid changes constantly throughout the month. Following your period, you will have a few days with little to no cervical fluid. I call this the dry spell. As your body gets ready for ovulation, your cervical fluid shifts to a rubbery consistency and is white or yellowish in tinge. Closer to ovulation, you may notice that the consistency becomes creamy. When estrogen levels finally surge, your cervical fluid becomes a viscous and stretchy egg-white-like substance known as *spinn*, from the German word *Spinnbarkeit*, meaning the ability to form a thread. That's your sign that ovulation is on!

Heed your cravings. Dietary choices can trigger or amplify physical symptoms, making us feel bad in some cases. Paying attention to physical indicators and their frequency and intensity can tell you when it might be a good idea to avoid certain foods like sugar, caffeine, dairy, corn, and wheat. Hydration and iron-rich, energy-boosting foods like goji berries, blueberries, trail mix, and leafy greens can get you through when you need a boost of improved focus while working. Your body will also tell you what types of foods it may need more of, like minerals, fats, proteins, and the beloved dark chocolate. Take note of what your body is asking for during each phase of your cycle. Do any patterns emerge?

Mind your mood. Your mood will shift, as your emotions are fluid throughout the cycle. Your interest in intimacy and sex will have peaks and valleys. If you notice you are feeling irritable or short-tempered on certain days, make time to be alone and take care of yourself. Note when you need to be surrounded by friends or when it feels good to cuddle up and watch Netflix and stay in. Don't force yourself to go out if you're not feeling up for it. Use this time to recharge.

Move your body. Movement energizes our cells, helps improve our mood, and even modulates our cravings. The exercise we partake in should change throughout the cycle. When bleeding, you may feel guilty that you are not exercising, but you may not feel like doing much of anything. It's important to honor that and allow yourself to stretch and to do light, grounding movements versus the high-impact movement that may feel great when you're ovulating. Don't be stubborn. Create variety in your workout routine; the same workout may not feel satisfying throughout the whole cycle. Sometimes a ballet class might be just what you needed instead of your usual kickboxing class. After a few months of mapping, you'll begin to know in advance what workouts will be best for which days.

Pay attention. Mapping your attention span, your creativity, and mental acuity can provide insight on how your mood and physical state may be enhanced or affected by your cycle. If you experience painful cramps and fatigue in connection with your period, you may not have the sharp attention span you're used to as compared to when you're not cramping. If you've put too much on your plate or you get a headache from the headiness of it all, take a break. Pay attention. Through mapping, you will be keenly aware of your needs for rest, naps, bedtime, and meditation.

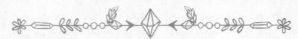

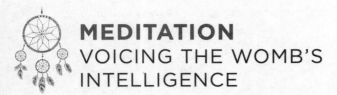

MEDITATION
VOICING THE WOMB'S INTELLIGENCE

Your body will tell you in no uncertain terms when it feels honored and safe or taken advantage of. Your body is the arbiter of what is safe, always. In any given situation in which you are exploring options, whether it's in the bedroom or the boardroom, I encourage you to tap into your womb's wisdom for the answer. Your power lies in the connection you have to the spirit door of your pelvis. The soul moves through the body, through the hips.

There is an ascension of energy that starts in the root of our beings and moves through the seven energetic portals in the body known as chakras, from the seat of the pelvis to the crown of your head. I'm asking you to stop trying to think your way through situations. Stop calling a lifeline for advice. Why not trust yourself, the one living and breathing within you, to help guide you to the answers?

Drop out of your head and into your womb and really ask yourself:

Does this feel right?

Do I truly want to do this?

Am I honoring my highest good by saying yes?

What mind-set do I need to lean into receive this?

When you are clear on what you want to happen for yourself, you can say yes, you can open up. Feel your way to the answers by tapping into your center of creativity. It all starts with what you feel within. Your wombifesting practice must include connecting with your womb chakra. You don't have to have a uterus in order to tap into this divine feminine energy; you can summon forth the creative matrix within you simply by acknowledging the power of the feminine and activating sacred womb intelligence through ritual.

Part of my self-care practice is using my voice daily. We are going to use your voice specifically as a healing instrument to send vibrations to your womb. We will practice a technique called "toning." Tone is an elongated pitch of sound. The mot comfortable range is closest to your speaking voice. The inhalations and exhalations are much longer when you are toning. It's an internal massage for your body that creates a vibration soothing to the nervous system. With toning, you create an extended vowel sound or syllable, usually with lips closed, like humming. It's not chanting or singing. It's simply holding a note continuously while letting the vibration of the sound resonate throughout your body and down to your womb.

Toning can help you get back in tune with your womb. Your voice is a powerful conduit of your intentions. When you set your intention for healing, toning delivers that healing vibration through the voice.

Lie comfortably on your back. Place your hands on your abdomen in the shape of a downward-pointing triangle. Close your eyes and relax your body. Deeply connect with this part of your body, ripe with potential. Receive a deep breath in, send healing warmth to your core, deep down into your womb. Exhale and release with a sigh. Continue breathing. On your next breath in, prepare to tone. Exhale and, with your lips closed, sound a steady pitch. Continue to tone consistently for five minutes. Then rest in silence and observe the resonance. Vibrational medicine is everything.

Connect with the living-feedback intelligence of your womb. Here is where the magic begins and is cultivated. Pray from this place, meditate from this place, dance from this place, create from this place, love from this place. This is the place you dwelled within your mother, and it's the place from which your hopes, dreams, ideas, and babies will come forth.

glow tips for
Wombifesting Your Wildest Dreams

Don't be afraid to ask. Claim what you want and ask for it. Place that request in a sacred space. If you keep an altar or have a personal space dedicated to prayer or meditation, go there and ask for the Universe to deliver and support you along the journey you so deeply desire.

Lean into vulnerability. Be open about your hopes and your failures. There is peace in being open and honest about who you are—your hopes, your triumphs, and your challenges. The most profound moments of inspiration happen when we get honest and allow ourselves to be naked. Whether you are giving a presentation at work, speaking on a stage, accepting an award, or calling in the love of your life, it requires vulner- ability—a softness of the heart and gaze—that you might see the world through warm eyes.

Seek moments of grace. A good way to be present in our bodies is to breathe mindfully, gently, and with compassion for others as well as ourselves. Draw out the best in yourself and everyone. Embrace the wilderness within yourself and scatter wildflower seeds. Look around you, always seeing the silver lining.

Cultivate openness. Openness allows learning to take place. Expose yourself to new ideas, read books that will challenge you to think differently, learn about other cultures and customs, and share these perspectives with your friends to stimulate honest dialogue. This will help to expand your consciousness as you wombifest.

Practice gratitude. Simply be in the practice of appreci- ating what you have going on right now without feeling the compulsion to compare, denigrate, or change the present.

Expect fluctuation. As the moon shifts on a daily basis, so do we. Sometimes you are going to be effective as your calm, receptive self, and other times, you will need to employ the part of you that is a lioness, a champion, a fierce mother. Protect yourself. It's okay to change your mind. When you come to understand that you are constantly changing and that what you feel will change, you will have an awakened understanding of your own internal flow and when to best tap into your most potent primal energy.

Awaken the body. Movement is the key to connection. Get out of your head and drop into your womb space. Rhythm, sound, movement, and breath united leads to trance. Using movement, stir up the magic within you. Dance, exercise, hiking, martial arts, anything that helps to create rhythmic movement in the hips, bringing blood flow and energy into your pelvis, is a good place to start.

Round up your vision doulas for support. Create a support system for where you are right now. In the birth tradition, the doula is a woman whose role is to "mother the mother." She is to serve as a grounding emotional and spiritual support for the woman who is transitioning, crossing a threshold into motherhood. Your vision doula holds the same role—to be an emotional and spiritual support for you while you hold space for something greater that is coming through you.

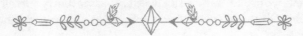

The symbolic manifestation of the great mother is the downward-pointing triangle—the source of dharmas, the cosmic cervix that is the gateway of all that is birthed. The triangle represents the feminine and the archetype of universal fertility. Sunyata, or "the void," is the primary creative matrix—the womb. The channel of the cosmic cervix, the great mother womb signifies the microcosm and macrocosm, the vastness of all things and the very little minutiae. Therein lies a miracle in your sacred anatomy. Woman, you are a living miracle. Are you not astounded at the magical, mystical, alchemical creation that is you? I'm grateful for the path of service that allows me to witness the living energy Universe emerge from the hips of women. I am grateful for the blessing of birth of all things and all it entails. Embrace your magic. Place your hand on your womb . . . Are you attuned?

personal process and prioritizing with passion

"I am learning every day to allow the space between where I am and where I want to be inspire me and not terrify me."

~ TRACEE ELLIS ROSS

The sacred feminine forces that we have uncovered here have an effect on all our processes. And our understanding and embrace of these forces can help us take steps toward bringing our mission into fruition. Taking steps on your journey toward transformation can be overwhelming, especially if you set your heart on some big life changes. But we've learned a lot about the greater feminine forces of the Universe and how we can use them to our advantage. Now it's time to explore your own individual best process. It's time to take your ideas and spin them into action. Now we own our strengths and embrace our growing edge—which is our most vulnerable blind spot. We want to learn how we work best and learn to trust in both our process and the Universe's timing. And, as part of that process, we need to prioritize our true purpose, to truly light a fire under ourselves so that nothing gets in the way of us living our best life.

We will celebrate our *only-ness* and learn about how the two hemispheres of our brain work and the balance of our feminine and masculine energies. We will learn how to practice patience with our goals and how to prioritize our mission. This chapter will help us tap into our unique gifts so that we can amplify them and share the best of who we are with others. When we know who we are and what we want, nothing can stop us.

There is something you want more than anyone else does. You're driven and have serious ambition and are known for creating or developing remarkable things that haven't been seen or done before. You not only think outside the box; you've decimated the box. You're a pretty pioneer out to explore what the world has waiting for you. You have a pure and fixed vision of what makes a difference, and you hustle to go get it. You seethe with impatience, yet you have some part of you that's open to hearing other opinions even when you *know* you're right. You are irreverent and beautiful, which means, by society's estimation, you're dangerous. It knows you're smart, witty, and can save the planet with your creative genius. You have a fierce energy pulsing through you that is matched by your unique talent. But you don't completely trust your process and rely heavily on the feedback of others to measure your value. You vacillate between feeling your power and needing approval.

Does this sound anything like you?

So, what are you waiting for, girl? Step outside of your coziest space. Extend yourself and shatter the barriers. Do things *your* way. Find and commit to your own process, your own method. It's fine to look to others for inspiration, but only you can create your blueprint for your success. Learn your strengths, learn to love them, and dial up that glow power full blast! Mapping your journey is a personal process, and I'm here to walk with you as you cross the river. Let's Glow!

Own Your Only-ness

Being who you are is celebrating the fact that there is only one you, so embrace your "only-ness." What makes you *you* is your unique genetic hardwiring and software—the things you've learned and downloaded along the way. Knowing your personality can guide you to the best environments for work, play, relationships, and recharging your batteries. Whatever your ultimate goal, understanding how your mind and body work can make the road to get there less of a struggle. You can prosper at home, work, and everywhere you go by increasing your connection with your unique self—owning your glow power and experiencing your life through a completely different lens. Business strategist and author Nilofer Merchant describes the term *only-ness* in her popular TED talk as "that thing that only one individual can bring to a situation." But it's not just a *thing*; your only-ness is a complex compilation of thought patterns, attitudes, feelings, and behaviors uniquely expressed by you. And when you know those quirks and kinks, rather than dismiss or subvert them, you can integrate them and use them to your ability.

Your unique personality impacts:

- How you respond to conflict and stress
- How you respond to times of transition
- How you create, innovate, lead, manage, and problem solve
- Your time-management and goal-setting styles
- How motivated you are
- How you prioritize

One of the greatest benefits of embracing your "only-ness" is increased self-acceptance. Embracing the fact that you carry a unique skill set onto the stage, a particular mix of traits that only you can offer to the world, makes accepting and owning these traits feel more natural. In a world where girls are told from a very young age that they are "not enough," it's so important to develop that self-acceptance and forgive what otherwise might be seen as our faults.

Too often, we have to convince ourselves that we are worthy of love, of success, and of fruitful relationships. The key is to understand and bolster your strengths and know your growing edge.

Find the optimal settings for your success. We know that plants need water, clean air, and sunlight to thrive and that the conditions have to be just so for the process to unfold smoothly. The same goes for us. We come encoded with a sacred mandate to live out our most powerful life—to live in the glow—and the right conditions can support our mandate, but we need to learn what they are and create a life that allows us to thrive, not just live. Understanding and accepting how you are hardwired will help you advocate for your needs and make intentional choices that set you up for success on this transformative journey. When we lift the veil of who we are supposed to be and start living our lives from a place of truth, compassion, divine connection, and community, then confidence and glow power will flourish.

The Battle of the Brains

I used to beat myself up all the time for working "out of order" and was often upset at myself for lacking the ability to focus on one thing at a time. I was frustrated by my appalling math skills. I'm left-handed and always felt like an outsider. It wasn't until I learned more about the brain and how distinctly each hemisphere processes information that I came to value my own process and to see that my differences are in fact reflective of my strengths.

The theory of the left and right brains, although often overgeneralized and oversimplified, can be used as a map to understand our innate strengths and how to better integrate both sides of the brain. The lateralization of brain function refers to how different processes and functions are located in one hemisphere or the other, and it's thought that in each individual, one or the other hemisphere might be dominant, leading them to possess certain strengths or attributes as opposed to those of someone whose other hemisphere dominates.

Right brain: According to left/right brain-dominance theory, the right brain is best at expressive and creative tasks. Popular abilities associated with the right brain include recognizing faces, expressing and reading emotions, musicality, sensing of color, seeing images, creativity, and intuition. These characteristics dominate the worlds of theater, fashion, architecture, music, mindfulness.

Left brain: The left brain is considered adept at tasks that involve logic and analytical thinking. The left brain's strengths include language, critical thinking, numbers, and reasoning. These are clearly characteristics that are valued in our global culture and standard business models.

I've delineated five relevant categories below for brain function and how they correlate across the left and right hemispheres. This is to help us start to see what our strengths are and where we may need to bolster our support.

	Information Processing	Project Engagement	Perception	Workflow	Problem Solving
Left Brain	Processes info in a linear manner	Identifies important details	Analytical, questioning	Sequentially, moves in order	Uses logic to solve problems
Right Brain	Processes info cyclically and holistically	Sees end result with clarity	Creative, abstract	Moves randomly from task to task	Uses intuition to solve problems

The beauty of this table is that it shows us the superpowers that each of our hemispheres holds. It turns out that I'm right-brain dominant, where a lot of the visioning and creative process we are exploring happens. (It also explains my left-handedness!) I'm someone who processes information holistically, so I need to write things down or draw and put them into sequential order when I delineate tasks for myself or others. I've learned to use some of the more linear tools (in this case, list making and keeping a planner) to help organize the more creative, organic process happening within me. Ideally we embrace this dynamic balance by celebrating our strengths and integrating the growing edge with outside support, either in the form of the tools available to us or the partners we choose to work with. Look at the table and see where your natural inclinations lie. How do you typically approach a problem? Do you tend to rush ahead, or are you a meticulous planner?

The unfortunate reality is that culturally, we undervalue the right brain's superpowers and prefer to deal with life in terms of direct, linear, sequential, analytical, logical process and outcome. Don't get me wrong! This is a valuable system because the objective or outcome is always tangible. This is how the world functions. But undeniably at the helm of any pursuit is a vision and creative concept that was brought to life using the skills employed by *both* sides of the dazzling brain.

According to Louann Brizendine, M.D., author of *The Female Brain*, "The female brain has tremendous and unique aptitudes—outstanding verbal agility, the ability to connect deeply in friendship, a nearly psychic capability to read faces and tone of voice for emotions and states of mind, as well as the ability to defuse conflict. All this is hardwired into the brains of women—these are talents that women are born with." When we understand that these abilities are what make us uniquely feminine and that they are accessible tools that help amplify our glow power, we can begin to embrace our visions and cultivate them with a totally new awareness. For my right-brained readers whose strengths are often downplayed, celebrate this natural inclination toward the creative. Left-brained readers, let's focus our work on tapping into those right-brain attributes that are within you that you might not naturally be inclined to exercise. There is an inherent strength that lies within you—let's amplify it.

Embracing Your Yin-ergy

In the same way that we must seek to achieve a dynamic equilibrium with regard to our cognitive processing, we must aim for that equilibrium with our dominant energies, embracing the feminine Yin energy that too many of us have suppressed in our efforts to survive in a male-dominated culture.

Most of my friends and many of the women included in these pages have hustled, been pioneers in their fields, and have made huge efforts to realize their dreams and goals. I encounter young women who are driven, focused, steady, and assertive. They know what they want, and they go and get it. This is admirable; however, it's not the only way to approach the path to success. So many of us have been conditioned to shut off our core feminine strengths to "get ahead," leading from our masculine energy.

In our work at Mama Glow, we've seen a rise in fertility challenges and female reproductive-related disorders in recent years that are directly correlated to lifestyle choices and stress. The stress that women experience in the workplace, compounded with the complexities of home life, responsibilities, and a lack of self-care, contribute to many of the reproductive issues that have surfaced in modern women. As a collective group, our connection to our total glow power and *yin-ergy* has been severed, and I believe that now it's critical to reconnect to our bodies and utilize our feminine strengths. I mean going underneath and exploring the principles that connect us to the cosmic order and using *that* to our advantage!

The Taoists understood that everything in our world is composed of two energies: Yin and Yang. These two fundamental forces complement each other and are both necessary for dynamic equilibrium—a living, breathing balancing act in our living energy universe. There are light and dark, night and day, hot and cold, sun and moon, feminine and masculine energies that govern everything. And each of these forces *and its complement* live within us. First, let's focus on the Yin. It is associated with the feminine—our core energy—and is aligned with the ever-fluctuating moon. It mirrors our ebbs and flows as women, from our hormonal shifts, our moods, and the fluctuations of our sexual arousal to the shifting energy of our menstrual cycles, pregnancy, birth, breastfeeding, and menopause. It's fluid, open, variable, and yielding. When yin is expressed, it is relaxed, open, secure, and receptive. Like water, yin is vast; it extends beyond the perimeters of the body, into the space between people. It is fueled by connection. Yin is process oriented, not focused on the outcome but enjoying the journey. Yin proceeds from the outside in; its energy is vast and creates a vacuum with which Yin draws things toward itself. It does not need to go out and get anything. Yet, it's not passive. That which it wants comes right to it. Yin energy is associated with wombifesting.

Yin magic is about transformation. Take the perfect act of pro-creation and conception, pregnancy, and birth. Yin receives the sperm and allows the egg to be fertilized and after 10 moons, a baby emerges. Magic. Your womb is a keeper of that very magic, that ability to alchemically create, transform, and give birth to golden, glowing new life, whether that be a child, a new business, a relationship, or a book. It is your yin-ergy at work when you *receive* inspiration, stir it up inside, and give birth to something new.

Everything starts at the seed level and grows in the darkness of the yin. The Universe is on our side. It's not about being "equal to men." The masculine is our complement, not our equal. And over-developing our masculine qualities while stifling our core feminine doesn't allow us to fully own our glow. Our job is to explore that dark yin space, to summon forth the creative matrix within and bring these aspects of ourselves and our gifts to the light. That is the act of standing in your glow power and embracing your yin-ergy.

RITUAL
YIN DARKNESS AND STILLNESS

Cultivate inner peace in the darkness. Darkness is a mystery unfolding that moves us toward the light.

Wake up just before the sun rises, when its dark, quiet, and still. Light a single candle, find a comfortable seat or lie on your back, and connect with your breath. As you sit in darkness, scan your body with your voice as a way to open and relax the body.

Stillness is a form of vibration and silence is a form of sound. Connect with the stillness, darkness, and silence. Listen to the ambient sounds of the early morning. Sit for a minimum of 15 minutes. Then close the ritual by setting an intention for your day and soul scribing for a few minutes while the sun rises.

Yang Complement

The yang energy is fast, fiery, focused. It's outward, active, and assertive. It is single pointed in focus, not a multitasking energy. It initiates and directs. Yang is associated with masculine attributes and qualities. Yang energy moves in and out, penetrating and withdrawing. It seeks to get to the center like an arrow to a bull's eye. Yang is impatient, insistent, and wants to get where it's going the quickest and most direct way possible.

You might be thinking, *Well, I have some of those* yinny *elements, but I know at my center I have some feisty, focused swagger that doesn't fall under the yin umbrella.* Well, you're right. We all have masculine elements of varying degrees that complement the feminine core. You may feel you are more dominant in your masculine energy and want to integrate more of the feminine. Sometimes, our complement overrides our core element, often creating inner conflict. Dual elements exist because of each other. The Yin needs the Yang to stay in balance, and vice versa. For example, Yin qualities include an outstanding ability to multitask and to see the big picture. But this multitasking quality can also permeate your boudoir, and you might find yourself easily distracted along the path of arousal. Have you ever been kissing and, during foreplay, started thinking about your to-do list instead? That's a time to pump up the laser focus of your yang complement and stay in the moment.

I don't want you to think you should not embrace your more traditionally masculine qualities. Yang attributes as a complement have some seriously useful benefits that can help us to round out our personal character and dial up our glow power. It's all about putting those qualities in balance and noticing where work can be done to accentuate your strengths, build the areas where you have a growing edge, and embrace the areas that need integration.

Yin-Yang Principles

Here is a list of the basic polar attributes of these dynamic energies. They mirror the qualities of the brain hemispheres that we discussed above.

YIN	YANG
Feminine	Masculine
Vagina	Penis
Cool	Hot
Watery	Fiery
Slow	Fast
Egg	Sperm
Inward	Outward
Wide focus	Single focus
Process-oriented	Goal-oriented
Receptive	Penetrative
Holistic	Fragmented
Sustains	Initiates
Subtle	Direct
Lunar	Solar
Fluctuating	Steady
Movement	Stillness
Cooperative	Competitive

Exploring Your Core Qualities

How would you describe your core qualities? Where could you use some softening? Where can you employ more Yin or Yang qualities? Take a look at the list below and identify the words that resonate most with your strengths. Then make a list of your top 10. You may come up with your own words that aren't listed. Then examine the words you chose—are they more yin or yang oriented?

Action-oriented	Athletic
Adventurous	Bossy
Aggressive	Caring
Analytical	Communicative
Artistic	Compassionate

Courageous	Optimistic
Determined	Organized
Disciplined	Outgoing
Emotional	Patient
Empathetic	Precise
Energetic	Self-controlled
Fast	Spontaneous
Flexible	Strategic
Focused	Team-oriented
Helping	Thoughtful
Inspiring	Visionary
Motivated	Warm
Open-minded	Wise

Process Makes Perfect

The Yin energy at our feminine core is process oriented, not out-come oriented. Despite what the world around us says, it's about the journey. That is one of the most important reasons for us to embrace and accentuate our yin-ergy. Being too outcome focused at the expense of fine-tuning the process can be truly destructive. The old adage is "practice makes perfect," but I believe that the key is not simply practice but process—engaging in something with our full attention—that makes perfect. And when I use the word *perfect*, I don't mean something flawless. I mean the divine incarnation of something that has gone from its beginnings to full blossom. An orange that has gone from flower to fruit and, now ripe, has swollen with sugars and fallen from the tree. Even if it is bruised or scarred from the fall, it is perfect. When we let process govern, the outcome is perfection.

So often, I work with women who jump around from project to project. First they have one idea they work on, then they switch to something else. Maybe the money isn't coming right away, or they get bored, or they don't want to put in the work but want the results. They end up with different things going on but nothing that has gone full term. If you're constantly switching directions, scrambling for the quickest way to reach a goal, that sends a message out into the ether that you're simply not ready. You're in fear mode, wanting the quickest solution to bring you comfort and security. The only way out is to go in, take the journey, and really do the work. We must learn to trust the process. That can be challenging for most of us, because we are so used to manipulating the process, trying to hustle and push things to move a certain direction to yield a specific outcome. But everything has its own divine timing, and it's not always in accordance with *our* schedules.

Sacred timing is all about readiness. When you are ready to move to the next level, you will be catapulted there, and not necessarily when you want it. Things don't happen when the time is right but when the timing is *ripe*. There is a timing that the Universe works with that has nothing to do with our schedules, our plans, or our agendas. Instead of trying to force things to move in a certain direction and expedite something that may take time to develop, just allow yourself to surrender to the process. When I work with expectant moms who are anxious to deliver their babies, I have to remind them that babies are born on their birthdays, not when it's convenient for us. Remember that human gestation takes 40 weeks, not 4 days. Everything takes time, and your time will come. Whether you are waiting to meet your life partner, waiting to make partner at your firm, or looking for the perfect partner to launch your new business with, do your part and leave the rest to the Universe to take care of for you.

However, honoring the Universe's timing does not mean sitting idly by. There are things we can do to move ourselves down the road toward achieving our ultimate goal. We've identified what it is we want to accomplish and what we want to call toward us, and we want to be sure to do the work so that when the Universe decides that the timing is right, we'll be ready to receive. That means doing what you can to make this mission, this life's purpose, your priority. Let's explore several different ways to cast a big, bright spotlight on your personal mission.

Multitasking vs. Uni-Tasking

How many times have you done just one thing at a time? Women are masterful multitaskers. With the über-busy, high-speed lives we lead these days, multitasking isn't simply the norm, it's the rule. I'm convinced that much of our modern stress is caused by a feeling that time is escaping us. We somehow feel the need to run to the place we are going, and we are racing through life just trying to get everything done in some impossible time frame. What type of life does that leave us living?

One really important lesson I've learned over time is to slow down and do one thing at a time. How can I possibly be productive if I am doing one thing at a time? How present are you when you are doing multiple tasks at once? If you allow yourself to do just one thing—from beginning to finish—limiting your external distractions, you actually do get *more* done. Focusing on one thing, bringing your attention to your intention, helps you stay the course and minimizes the feeling of perpetual overwhelm. My friend Arianna Huffington, founder of Thrive Global and *New York Times* best-selling author of *The Sleep Revolution*, says that multitasking is the downfall of modern society. Do the easiest things first, the things that feel pleasurable to do, because you will accomplish these tasks with ease and efficiency and without much effort.

Uni-tasking in action. I know it's not easy to do one thing at a time when you can do three, but uni-tasking means that rather than cooking dinner while talking on the phone and watching TV, you leave your phone on the charger and prepare a healthy meal with total concentration, love, and awareness. The art of uni-tasking allows me to read a book to my son as he prepares for bed, making us both feel more relaxed as we wind down for the night. It's in our nature to be able to juggle so many things, but with the speed at which we live, it feels good to slow it down. When we think about what we are missing out on, it turns out that it's usually the present moment. Surrender is not giving up; it's giving over. It's letting go, releasing. Slow down, listen, and reconfigure your to-do list accordingly so that you punctuate your life with the artful skill of uni-tasking.

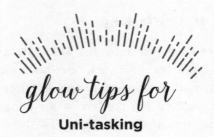

glow tips for
Uni-tasking

Prioritize. Figure out what you need in your schedule personally and professionally and what you can legitimately take off your plate. What are the top three things you need to get done today?

Delegate. What systems and people need to be in place for you to offload some of your duties, and which of those duties can you completely give over to someone else to manage for you?

Set boundaries. Establish some really clear boundaries to operate by, and set a standard for when you shut off work mode.

Phone-fast. Once a week, for a partial or full day, get off the phone and all electronics. Stop texting, checking Instagram, and all your feeds. Stay focused on your internal status.

Get present. Take a look at how you are actually spending your time. You want to be investing your time in memories and enjoying your life, not simply crossing off things on your to-do list and paying bills. I invite you to really start being mindful of the moment. Breathe deeply. Yes, you could be in a million other places right now, but you are here, so *be* here.

Stir It Up!

When your energy is focused on the mundane tasks of day-to-day living, oftentimes, your passions can get shelved. And most of the time, you don't even consciously realize that you've put your joy on hold. Do you recall a time as a child when your big-time aspirations were normal and everything seemed possible? You didn't know how to do it all, but you knew it was possible, because you could envision it.

When the years start stacking and responsibilities pile up and when commitments to work, family duties, and financial constraints require more of your attention, your soul voice becomes overcast by the fear and trepidation that you must "make it happen." Before you know it, you've shut the door on yourself and can't seem to get clear on what you want in life, because all you can focus on is making ends meet.

Does this sound familiar? Do you believe it's true? Do you believe that if you are following the path intended for you that you will be called upon to do things you don't want to do? I believe that when we are given situations that appear to have a single and bleak outcome, it's an opportunity to rise up, dive into our creativity, and stir up a solution from within.

Many of my friends lost their jobs during the 2008 financial crisis, and while some of them wallowed in self-pity, downsized their lifestyles, and slowly spent their savings, others thrived. My friend Tiffany, who had been a lawyer, reignited her passion for baking. She had always loved to bake as a hobby, but suddenly, with all the time she had, there was an opportunity for her to grow a business—one that proved to be lucrative—her famous red-velvet cupcakes spiked with Rémy Martin were a hit. It was because she had been dealt a "bad hand" that she realized that she had the solution within. She could fall back on her passion.

The good news is, you don't need to leave it to the Universe completely. You can acknowledge your purpose now, own the dream you've decided on, and make it a priority today. There are many reasons that we don't prioritize our life's purpose. If we haven't set clear intentions, then we might not know what we're reaching for. Maybe we're crystal clear on what we want, but we're keeping it to ourselves instead of putting it out there in the world. Or maybe we're overwhelmed by the enormity of the undertaking, and so we don't take that first fateful step. Let's solve those problems now. Let's make this transformation you're seeking a reality. Let's make this mission a priority so that the Universe will see just how ready you are.

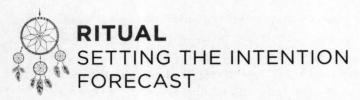

RITUAL
SETTING THE INTENTION FORECAST

The first step in prioritizing is knowing exactly what we're reaching for and seeing it in front of us. I want you to set some crystal-clear intentions; your focus needs to be laser sharp. If you're a bit unsure or on-the-fence about what you want, baby, you may find that the results you get are equally as unclear. Clarity is potent, and its charge is electric, which means it carries a message or thought farther and to its desired target. If you're seeking new love, you want to be clear on exactly what kind of support you need from a partner. If it's a new job you're seeking, you should be able to visualize yourself in that space, doing the exact work you desire and succeeding at it.

When you write your intentions, frame them in the positive present tense. We are holding the archer's bow, and with steadiness and a single-pointed gaze, we are aiming to hit the bull's eye. When the archer holds the bow and gazes upon the target that may be over a hundred feet away, she sees the arrow cutting the wind and bending ever so slightly to reach its destination, one that was already mapped out with precision. It's already done, even though the arrow has yet to be released. So when we speak in the present tense, we are acknowledging that something is already done. We have seen it. Intention actualizes potential. Your intention forecast statements might sound something like:

- *I am sitting on my terrace along the beach in Northeastern Brazil, writing my screenplay, and I'm filled with joy.*

- *My business is thriving, I am signing five new clients monthly and generating $200,000 annually.*

- *I am holding my blossoming pregnant belly, blissfully happy, and married to the man or woman of my dreams.*

- *I am loving my new apartment overlooking the river and am enjoying a perfect sunset on the rooftop with friends, and I am grateful.*

- *I am comfortable in my own skin, having lost the weight of my past emotions and poor habits, and embrace a healthy figure and wardrobe full of clothes that express and reflect who I am.*

Shout, Shout, Let It All Out!

Now that we've visualized and set our intentions, it's time to amplify them! Amplify your dream by sharing it. Talk about it! Be about it. Shout it from the rooftops! Tell people about your big dream, because when you do, you breathe life into your vision. You catapult yourself beyond intention and into action, creating an environment of accountability that'll support your growth and keep you on your toes. Plus, you build a network of cheerleaders who want to see you win *and*, since everyone knows what you are looking to achieve, you build a conscious network of potential supporters—people who start to believe in your dream and become invested in seeing you bring it to life. These people may be mentors, financial supporters, board members, or people who connect you with potential opportunities that help you along the way. Now, I know there are people that do not deserve to hear what you have to share, so use discernment and open up to those who offer you a safe space.

What about those who may steal my ideas? If you are concerned about people who might steal your ideas, then you are investing in a belief system rooted in scarcity. There are more ideas where the ones you have came from, and the bottom line is that there is only one you, and only you can do what you do. Even if anyone tries, they won't be able to do it like you can. Yes, you should protect your intellectual property, but you shouldn't worry about who's out there trying to copy you. What's meant for you is yours and yours alone. Trust and believe that others can never be you. Keep going and don't let the stifling fear of people stealing your ideas keep you from bringing your important message to the world.

The Juju Is in the Momentum

Now you have cheerleaders behind you. Feel their breath at your back as you move forward and don't be daunted by the enormity of this undertaking. Baby steps lead to quantum leaps. Being energetically aligned with your dream, determined, and consistent in your actions ultimately creates change. Don't stop; keep taking steps forward. You don't have to know where you are going. Just give yourself permission to put one foot in front of the next and keep walking.

So, will you make that phone call? Will you write that email you've been putting off? Will you put up that blog post that you have been too nervous to share? Will you sign up for that enrichment workshop that you are terrified of or join the group fitness class you think you're not good enough for? Will you take the opportunity to speak up for yourself, to seek out a mentor, to allow your curiosity to override fear so that you actually enroll in the course? Will you ask your boss for a reduction in hours because you are openly pursuing your quest, your passion project? Will you do that for yourself? Will you just give yourself permission?

WILL YOU FOCUS ALL YOUR ENERGY ON BUILDING THE SHINY NEW STUFF OF YOUR DREAMS?

Quickly list five things you could do this week to move closer to your dream.

Make a passion promise to yourself that you will act on every one of these small, right actions to work toward your goal because you deserve to live a passionate, juicy life!

Get Help!

When I say to get help, I'm not talking about therapists, necessarily. I mean find someone who is excited to get their hands dirty and get into your vision and what it takes to bring it to life. Oftentimes when we hit a road block, our momentum takes a nosedive. Don't let that happen to you! Find someone to help you over that hurdle!

Does data entry make you crazy? Do spreadsheets drive you mad? Is it graphic design that would take your work to the next level or a person who is savvy with tech that could make a huge difference in the next phase of your business? Draft an email to your closest, most ambitious, and inspiring friends, and ask if they know anyone who meets your criteria for a professional soul mate. Stay in your zone of inspiration and outsource the rest. Perhaps seek the support of a life coach to help you get organized as you meet your new personal goals.

Cultivate a Passion Practice

Listening to your deepest desire to tap into your passion and glow power doesn't come effortlessly, particularly with the competing influences in our busy modern lives. You have to prioritize your passion. There are some distinct qualities that will make your creative journey more focused and consistent, which will in turn lead to increased satisfaction and joy in all areas of your life.

Discipline. Be your own disciple. Motivate yourself to stay aligned with what you most desire, tap into the skills and your unique gifts that will contribute to your success. Show up every day, committed to help move the process along.

Devotion. You may be devoted to your meditation practice, your gratitude journal, or your morning cup of coffee. Your morning devotion observance should be about play— draw, play music, dance to your favorite pop song, or practice yoga. Devote yourself to your passion.

Determination. Maintain a firm sense of purpose and resolve in your personal strength to keep steadfast to the vision and passion that animates you. This tenacity will ignite a spirit of strength to get you beyond self-doubt and procrastination.

Desire. What is the longing feeling inside leading you to? What do you aspire to create in this wild life of yours? What feelings are aligned with the visions you are bringing to life?

What words embody those feelings? Write them down and seek to feel them throughout your day.

Divine delight. Spread your beauty and joy to others by spreading bliss and living in your glow power. When you give yourself permission to create, you will become enchanted, inspired, fascinated, and cosmically tied to that passion, and you will captivate and inspire others.

RITUAL
DAILY DEVOTION

Today, devote yourself to your own creativity with dedication and divine discipline. Take out your journal and colored pens or pencils. Write some words of intention about your current desired agenda. Then add color to your words in whatever way feels good. Make a commitment to do a page each day centered around your passion pursuit. Make sure you spend some good time focusing on these five principles and incorporating them into your life. You may want to put Post-it notes or posters on the wall with these words and actions, life experiences, and quotes that help you stay tapped into these passion principles.

glow tips for
Making Your Passion a Priority

Set daily reminders in your phone. *Passion playtime starts now!* This will ensure that you make time for what you're aiming for.

Affirm your dreams. Cover your office/computer/fridge/bathroom mirror/corkboard/bedroom door with Post-its scrawled with positive affirmations. Let's call them Zen Notes. I like to think of BET's *Being Mary Jane,* where starlet Gabrielle Union's character, Mary Jane, lives in a sea of Post-it notes.

Declare your goals to your personal community. Your courage to start a dream accountability group is a crucial step toward prioritizing your passion. This can be a secret forum, a mastermind group, a coaching group, or an online community that holds you accountable to your goals.

MEDITATION
FREE MOVEMENT

Find a piece of music that inspires you and evokes a feeling you want to embody. Sit up tall on a chair, or stand. Gently close your eyes. Receive three long, deep, full breaths. Inhale and sweep your arms up over your head, and exhale while bringing your arms down alongside your body. Do this three times.

Place your hands onto your heart.

Turning your vision inward, receive a deep breath, and let your gaze travel down to your heart. See it glowing from within. What color do you see in your mind's eye?

You are creating an even bigger vibrational field around your heart, expanding its capacity for love, for compassion to yourself, and for the devotion you have to your goals. As you inhale, imagine yourself as a tree rooting your feet deep into the earth's soil and with your arms extending up toward the sky.

Soften your elbows so that your arms create a cradle overhead. You are in a receptive posture open for the wisdom, inspiration, and flow of ideas.

As the wind blows, the tree sways. Allow your upper body to sway with the breeze, making circular motions with your arms and torso.

Feeling rooted in the soil through your legs and feet, imagine the next iteration of your life unfolding before you. Every aspect of your life is nurtured by the nutrient-dense soil and natural elements.

Allow the swaying to turn into full-body movement. Take 10 minutes to explore dynamic movement with your eyes softened or closed. Allow yourself to move beyond your seat or standing area where you have freedom to—onto the floor, into the hallway. Allow the movement to govern your body. Surrender to the movement.

If you don't feel as inclined to move freely and you're struggling through this piece, turn on your favorite upbeat song and put it on repeat. Begin to dance!

"No matter where you stand right now—on a hilltop, in a gutter, at a crossroads, in a rut—you need to give yourself the best you have to offer in this moment. Rather than depleting yourself with judgments, redirect that energy toward the next big push—the one that takes you from enough to better. The one that takes you from adequate to extraordinary. The one that helps you rise up from a low moment and reach for your personal best."

- Oprah Winfrey

MOTIVATION MIX TRACK:
"THE GOSPEL" by Alicia Keys, *Here*

portal no. 3

EMBODY

embody |em'bädē|

verb: to be an expression of or give a tangible or
visible form to (an idea, quality, or feeling)

• to provide (a spirit) with a physical form.

• to include or contain (something)
as a constituent part

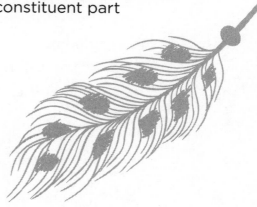

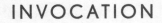

INVOCATION

~

Flanked in Red rose petals
Draped in perfumed golden silk robes
Undulating like water
Love Adorned
Bejeweled with grace
Perched upon a
Pedestal she built for
Herself
Majestic
Under sovereign rule of
Her soul
Crowned
In her own glory
Ascension
She knows she is worthy
Gaze fixed upon her light within
Behold
The Glow

~

reclaiming your queendom

"Here in this body are the sacred rivers. I have not encountered another temple as blissful as my own body."

~ FROM THE TEACHINGS OF THE SARAHA DOHA, ONE OF THE FOUNDERS OF THE BUDDHIST VAJRAYANA

After learning about feminine forces, best individual process, prioritizing the work, and trusting the process, we keep the momentum and enter the Embody portal. This is where you rise and become a woman living her best life. Maintain the trajectory of this transformative journey by reclaiming your queendom—standing firmly in your glow power, putting yourself first through radical self-care, self-acceptance, and owning your style. We learn how to find support through mentorship and how to be great mentors, how to build friendships in accountability, trust, and guidance, as well as how *to be* that guide for someone else.

I once had the privilege of hearing the legendary actress and recording artist Diahann Carroll speak about her illustrious career as one of the first African-American leading ladies on screen, and she told a story about meeting with a director that stuck with me. This particular director was one she had very much wanted to work with, and she spoke of how she'd adorned herself in her finest Givenchy and pearls in preparation for their meeting at the Plaza Hotel. When she arrived, she immediately spotted the director in his seat, but she did not acknowledge him. Instead, she allowed *him* to discover *her*. As his eyes fell upon her, he observed her grace, beauty, and elegance and was taken aback. Ms. Carroll then made eye contact, and, in that moment, she realized something. "When I looked at him, I knew he recognized that I am someone who knows that I am special, and I don't allow anyone to think otherwise."

That attitude alone, never mind her tremendous talent, would have allowed Diahann Carroll to bust through barriers and make history. She believed in and embraced her glow power and still does. She doesn't hide the very things that make her feminine; she amplifies them. Diahann Carroll carries herself in such a regal way, with her head held high. She thinks about how she wants the world to perceive her. It's not just about the dress and pearls but the love for herself that she exudes. She firmly stands in her queendom.

We are always saying that we want to be treated like queens. And the best way to get someone to treat you like a queen is to act like one—gaze through queenly eyes and walk the earth like it's your dominion. For some of us, it takes a bit of role playing; we may not feel as comfortable sporting our crowns because of the stories we may still be carrying about ourselves. Growing up in a global culture that finds fault with women at every turn has a way of permeating one's consciousness. We have collectively bought into the idea of playing small, but we can also decide to play big, to rebuff the dominant view of women.

You must stand in your queendom and own your glow. You can light the way not only for yourself but for women coming behind you who are also seeking to step into their authentic power. When we choose to play the role of one who is powerful, we embody its power, and suddenly we can harness the energy necessary to catapult us further in our lives.

So, how do we reclaim our queendom and amplify that glow power? We're ready for the next step on our journey, the Embody portal. It's all about being *selfish*. By putting yourself first, you can maintain optimal wellness in mind, body, and spirit. Ask yourself, "What would the queen within do in my situation?"

Treat yourself like a queen; truly embodying that royal persona means focusing on radical self-care. Self-care is a catalyst for transformation. You're on a divine mission, and you can't forget about your own well-being while birthing your vision and setting your goals ablaze. We'll need to practice self-acceptance, learning to love our bodies and affirm our reflections. We have to speak affirmations and blessings to ourselves daily. The more we develop a healthy inner balance, the likelier we are to be drawn to partners who are healthier, too. The more you romance yourself, the more you prepare yourself to be romanced. And, like Ms. Carroll, we'll own our style and our femininity and find joy in dressing for the life we want as we reclaim our royal queendom.

Reclaim Self-Care

Self-care is a critical aspect of reclaiming your queendom. We need to protect ourselves by erecting boundaries, not to trap ourselves inside, but to allow ourselves to filter what we allow into our lives. Pampering, or what I call *glow time,* is an opportunity to practice loving ourselves, to improve our relationship with our bodies and honor our physical needs. Intimacy can be a fulfilling aspect of our lives, and love and sexuality can help fuel our passion for our mission. What follows will be a journey into the specific ways in which we can take care of ourselves.

Create Royal Boundaries

You need to be able to distinguish between what to allow into your realm and what needs to stay outside your palace gates. Create boundaries in the workplace, at home, and in relationships. Women have inherited a legacy of taking on more than we can handle; we must activate the power of the word *no*. Pleasing others at the expense of ourselves is a habit that you will challenge while doing this work and beyond. It's your life and it must be *full* of joy, not just punctuated with fleeting moments of joy. Practice saying no. Start small.

Maybe there is a dinner that you would rather not attend but feel obligated to. Politely decline. Do not give an excuse; simply say, "Thank you for the invitation, but I will not be attending." Stop apologizing for saying no. It's okay if it makes others uncomfortable; it's not about preserving their feelings while yours are compromised. Saying no more often actually allows you the freedom to say yes to the things you should be doing more of, the things you love. You don't have to hold on to a commitment or resentment. Only say yes to what inspires you!

Sometimes we need to create boundaries with ourselves as well, because we need to unlearn old habits. Do not sacrifice sleep, manicures, or meals. Do not sacrifice your time to someone who saps your energy. Are you someone who stays on the phone and listens to a friend drag on and on about how she got into a huge argument with a lady at the post office? If you hang up the phone and then need a yoga class just to get your mind and spirit right, then your friend is probably someone you need to draw some boundaries with. Where do you need to put walls up? Who might be a good accountability partner, one who helps you stay on track and reminds you to honor your boundaries?

Glow Time

Every queen needs her time for royal relaxation, and I'm the queen of glow time, which is a self-care movement. It's about unapologetically choosing yourself first and recharging through rituals. My self-care practice helps me stay on course. Even my busiest days are fueled by a strong self-care practice. When we indulge ourselves in self-care on a regular basis, we allow self-renewal, healing, and restoration. Whether it's a weekly massage, a royal foot rub, a mini-facial, a glass of wine with a good piece of dark chocolate, curling up with a good book, getting your hair blown out, doing what makes you feel amazing is essential for your well-being.

Obviously, the list of what you can indulge in to please yourself is lengthy. But how often do you *really* indulge in your own self-care? When you practice glow time is also important. Whether you make it a regular occurrence, not just an occasional treat, is up to you, but I recommend creating a ritual that becomes part of your routine.

You may feel guilty taking time for yourself. But it's crucial to claim your glow time; nobody else will give it to you.

Your glow, by the way, is not for anyone else but you. It's not so your hair, nails, or lashes look good for some guy or girl. It's about mapping this time for yourself on your calendar and committing to your personal glow-time routine and making it a part of your life. And when pampering yourself at home, use the cleanest products you can find. Your skin is your largest organ, so you want to fortify yourself with the good stuff only.

What's essential to glow time is that it constitutes an alternative to everything that is fast and spinning in our lives. You cannot practice glow time while stressed out or in a hurry, as it is the art of creating intimacy with yourself, which can only be achieved through slowing down and mindfulness. The Danish lifestyle concept of *hygge,* which means "to comfort," encapsulates a mood, well-being, and feeling of being embraces and is the pinnacle of glow time. Glow time is about feeling safe.

GLOW-TIME PRINCIPLES

Atmosphere and mood. Considering the space and make adjustments for comfort first. This includes lighting, temperature, color, sounds, and scent.

Presence and pleasure. Being in the present moment, cutting out the noise of our lives, and experiencing the magic of the mundane feeds the soul. Whether you're hiking, having a summer picnic, or relaxing for movie night, pleasure is in the present moment.

Comfort and coming together. Glow time offers a way to be social that is not draining. Gathering with a small rather than a huge group of people is a way to nourish yourself. Even when you're alone, it's important not to feel isolation. When individuals experience social isolation, many of the same areas of the brain are active as when one is experiencing physical pain. Feeling a sense of belonging is key. The art of glow time is about expanding your comfort zone to include others.

Grace and gratitude. Happiness is directly correlated to our sense of gratitude. Count every little blessing because every blessing counts! Taking time regularly to reflect on the grace and abundance in your life will increase your happiness and keep the blessings flowing.

Slowing down and savoring. Accelerated living often keeps us from savoring the sweetness of life's precious moments. When we slow down to watch the snow fall, sip a cup of tea, and smell the flowers, we savor the present moment.

Establish a Royal Glow-Time Routine

Let's figure out what makes the most sense for your active schedule and use your calendar to map out what you want to include. This is not optional; it's obligatory. You will thank yourself! Have fun with it!

- How much time will you allot to yourself? An hour a day? Or 30 minutes each night?
- What are some feel-good practices you can incorporate into your schedule? Let's brainstorm.
- At what time of you day do you feel most constrained, and what do you usually do about it?
- When will you start implementing your glow-time routine?

Reclamation Rituals

Sometimes our glow time takes the form not just of routine, but of ritual. Rituals are powerful symbolic experiences that can be both simple and life-changing. They can incorporate the gifts of Mother Nature—oils, water, plants, and stones—and offer peace, tranquility, and can help us reclaim a sense of inner glow. Ritualistic practices provide inner strength, and there are simple rituals we can adopt that promote well-being and optimal health. Taking a hot bath and lathering on coconut oil or drinking a warm cup of tea to wind down in the evening are ways we might engage in simple rituals.

Creating your own ritual practice is easy. Start with identifying what brings you serenity each day. Treat yourself to a moment of silence; curiosity seeds your consciousness when the mind can be still. Perform a sacred act each day that means something profound to you and use that act to harness your glow power and ground you in peace within. Mundane routines like making your bed each morning can be *made* to be ritual when we perform them with a certain intention or mindfulness.

How we start and end our day matters and can determine our overall mood. Rituals performed at these times make space for much-needed mindfulness. The slowness allows us to tune in and become reflective. Rise up and go to bed mindfully. The morning is the beginning of a new day, a fresh start, and evenings are a time to reflect on the intention for the next day and hold space for gratitude for the robust day we have co-created.

Suggestions for Glow-Time Rituals

- **Morning Tonic.** Purify your body with hot water and lemon.
- **Fortify Your Body.** Have a breakfast smoothie.
- **Sacred Scent.** Use essential oils and flower essences.
- **Take It to the Head.** Headstands and handstands can clear your mind.

- **Light Candles.** Say your prayers or meditate.

- **Soul-Scribing.** Journal or write affirmations.

- **Prance and Dance.** Blast your favorite playlist, close your eyes, and dance like no one is watching.

- **Bathtub Time.** Soak it out and chill out.

- **Home Spa.** Practice a green beauty routine at home.

- **Solo Sex.** Caresses, touches, and intimacy alone are a healthy pathway to loving yourself.

- **Nap Time.** Naps are incredible and highly underrated. The siesta is back.

- **Nook Time.** Retreat to a small space. Tiny spaces often bring us comfort because they remind us of the small caves our ancestors once inhabited to keep safe.

- **Ground yourself in the Garden.** Join a community garden or create a garden of your own.

- **Soak Up the Sun.** Lie out in sunshine or take a morning walk with the early sun.

- **Write a Letter.** Once a week, write a card to someone you adore.

- **Bloom Your Room.** Keep fresh flowers in your line of vision.

- **Create your Glow Time Kit.** Put together a Glow Time kit that includes plain or scented candles, dark chocolate, herbal tea, your favorite book or movie, cozy socks, pajamas, a soft blanket, music, massage oil or moisturizing cream, essential oils, and a fuzzy hoodie.

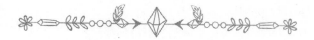

VIRIDESCENT MATCHA BATH TRUFFLES

These glorious green matcha bath truffles make for a lush bath-time experience. They are incredibly easy to make at home and are great glow time gifts.

What you will need:

- 3 cups baking soda
- 1 cup citric acid
- 2 tablespoons matcha
- 1 teaspoon liquid chlorophyll
- 1 cup Shea butter, melted
- 1 bath bomb mold
- 1 teaspoon witch hazel
- 5 drops sandalwood oil
- 5 drops vanilla oil

Directions:

Combine the baking soda and citric acid in a large bowl.

Add the matcha, green chlorophyll, Shea butter, sandalwood oil, and vanilla oil.

Spray the molds with witch hazel.

Once the bath truffle mixture has reached a moldable consistency, fill half of the mold with the matcha mixture, and set aside.

Slightly overfill the other half of the mold with the rest of the mixture and squeeze the two halves of the mold together.

Allow to set for 20 minutes, then gently twist and pull one half of the mold away.

Once one half of the mold is removed, leave the truffle in the mold to harden and gently remove the other half of the mold.

Allow the truffles to harden for at least 24 hours before putting to use.

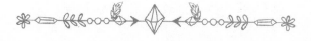

glow tips for

Self-Care and Managing Your Balancing Act

Ask for help. Every queen knows that it takes a royal court to help facilitate all the happenings within her queendom. The queen doesn't do it all alone. Remember to ask for help and practice the art of delegation. We feel so uncomfortable asking others to help us, but we need to realize that we can do more and better when we have support.

Take a nap. That's right, nap time is no longer for toddlers. It's a very useful wellness tool. When we take naps, we create space for our dreams. We allow the body to recover from the stress of our day. If you're too busy during the week to take an 8-to-20-minute nap, set aside some time on the weekend to tuck yourself into your bed or find a nice cozy resting space and catch some Zs.

Be a friend. Cherish your friends. Having a good friend to lean on for support is important for your mental and emotional well-being. Having someone to talk to, confide in, and share hopes, dreams, laughter, secrets, and support with is a blessing. If you want to have a friend, you must be a friend. You never know what your friends may be going through. Pick up the phone and tell your friends how much you love them. Make plans for a visit, take a hike together, or go to yoga class.

Soak it out. A mixture of Dead Sea salt, Epsom salts, essential oils like lavender, and hot water is the perfect ending to a long day. To really do it big, treat yourself to a nice scented candle or two. Shut off the phone and the lights and relax in the tub for a minimum of 15 minutes. Soaking detoxifies your cells, soothes tense muscles, and puts your mind at ease, too.

Get up and glow. Exercise during the mornings whenever possible. When you move your body at the start of your day, it decreases your appetite and stimulates the thyroid to burn calories all day long. Try power yoga, walking, jogging, swimming, or spinning, and add some resistance training at the end of the workout to further stimulate the fat-burning process. This might include push-ups, pull-ups, crunches, and squats. Or, instead of a morning gym routine, you could do some of the things you love outdoors in the early-morning sunshine, like Rollerblading, bike-riding, recreational sports, dancing, or walking. When you do what you love, you're happiest. It's exercise without the effort.

Hug Someone. Stress is the body's response to perceived threat. The emotional effects of stress include lack of forgiveness, distrust, and lack of intimacy. Negative thoughts can activate stress. The antidote to stress is breathing since it elicits the relaxation response. Hugging is therapeutic medicine; it calms the nervous system and induces the relaxation response. If the embrace lasts at least 20 seconds, the neurotransmitter oxytocin is released, creating an increased sense of bonding. If there is no one around for you to hug, cuddle up under a weighted blanket to feel swaddled and supported.

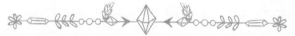

Embrace Intimacy

Embracing intimacy and soulful connection is an important aspect of self-care and reclaiming your queendom. Tuning in to pleasure and allowing yourself to experience vulnerability accentuates your glow. Relationships are a gift for personal growth and help us along the transformative journey we are taking. If you have found love, you have been given one of life's greatest gifts. We are not meant to move through this experience alone but with someone else. And if we want to change our relationships for the better, we have to examine ourselves first. That starts with making space for true intimacy. Most traditions call intimacy "surrender." Intimacy threatens our agency, and so we become guarded to protect our most tender asset, our hearts. But opening to intimacy is crucial nonetheless.

It is when you are loved and in love that you become highly perceptive and capable of seeing truth and light. My partner's love has helped me see more light; it hasn't blinded me but has given me super vision and inspired me. Love is a vehicle for growth, and it is the duty of the beloveds to draw the best from one another and dive deep to create something beautiful together. What will our sacred contribution be together, to each other, and unto the world? Where will we go and what will we do to transform ourselves through love? Through tiny acts of daily kindness and challenges met with grace, we rise and become the best lovers for each other. I will do my best to rise up and become who I need to be to serve my lover, my partner, my friend. I have learned to open to love.

Setting the Bar for Love vs. Settling for Less

When my single clients come to me about wanting to start a family but haven't yet found the partner they seek, I often recount to them the story of one of my dearest friends. She and I went to dinner at an upscale restaurant. We are both particular about food—asking the waiter to swap certain ingredients for others, concocting vegan masterpieces of our own that can't be found on the menu—and when her main course arrived, she took one bite, rolled her eyes, dropped her fork, and produced a frown like no other. She said, "I can't eat this; it's way too salty." The server rushed over when he caught her gaze, and she began to list what was wrong with her meal. She sent it back. Minutes later, the server brought out a different plate that completely met her standards, and she was happy.

As we ate, we talked about life, love, work, and relationships, and, in the midst of her monologue about her subpar love life, I was having a hard time focusing. I couldn't believe the same woman who had just been so clear and decisive about her standards for cuisine was so *unclear* about her standards for romance. She was making all sorts of excuses for a man who wasn't showing up in the way she wanted. My ears needed a break. "Pause," I said. "You just sent back a plate of food because it didn't meet your expectations, but you're telling me you are settling for this *shitty* relationship? Is that what we're doing right now? Settling? How does that make any sense?"

My friend isn't alone. Many of us will send back a cold plate of pasta but take what we think we can get when it comes to dating and relationships. We don't call out behavior that is inappropriate, and we involve ourselves in drawn-out love tangles with people who haven't proven worthy of our time, energy, or breath. Our standards should be consistent across the board—we shouldn't lower the bar to accommodate anyone, no matter how cute, accomplished, or amazing in bed. If a man wants to be with you, he will do what it takes to make you feel safe, precious, respected, and loved.

I hear so many women say, "This guy is eighty percent of what I want. He is so great. *But* . . ." or, "All the good ones are taken." The truth is, all the "good ones" aren't taken; they just are not visible to women locked into low vibration or scarcity consciousness. There are a ton of men and women out there who are seeking their divine reflection in partnership. But we can only see people operating on the same vibration; we can only see at the level of consciousness that we are open to. When we hold ourselves in high regard, the men that we once saw are no longer visible, and the men whom we couldn't see before, we can suddenly see in abundance. We open ourselves up to a whole new world of "good ones."

All this applies to women in same-sex relationships as well. Hold your partner or your prospect to a high-enough standard. When you expand your love for yourself and become what you seek in someone else first, then your scope for a quality person and relationship will increase. You need to step out the gate with a sense of fulfillment in your own life before you begin to engage romantically with someone else so you are not dependent upon him or her for your happiness. It is not a man's (or woman's) job to make you happy; that's your job. But it is your partner's job to *keep* you happy.

"Remember: Your self-regard sets the bar for all of your relationships. If you insist you are unworthy, you'll inevitably populate your life with those who agree."

- Terri Cole,
Real Love Revolution

glow tips for

Raising the Bar and Increasing Love in Your Life

Speak up with your actions, not just your words. We often speak about what we want and how we want to be treated, but the embodiment of these powerful words speaks volumes. If you want to be taken seriously, carry yourself that way. Don't just talk about it; *be* about it. If you're asked out on a date at the last minute, you can politely decline and assure the requester that you'd love to go when it's planned with advance notice. Commit to yourself first.

Stop dating for distraction. Don't use dating as an excuse to avoid your own personal soul work. It's easy to go out with someone because they are in your orbit, but make sure you are ready and interested, not just bored or lonely.

Solo date. Take time to date and fall in love with yourself. Treat yourself to gifts and getaways. Find a class that you would do with a partner and do it alone instead. Go to a romantic dinner with yourself. *Make* a romantic dinner for yourself. This is a glow time practice that will expand your glow.

Mind your feelings. Feelings don't lie. Whenever your body speaks to you, listen. Usually these gut feelings—butterflies or queasiness—are telling you something. The answer is either yes or hell no. When you are feeling a sense of doubt, go inward and investigate. Your intuition is designed to protect you and keep you thriving.

Let him call. All my hunter goddesses out there are probably getting anxiety when reading this, but as much as we think that times have changed, we still operate from a primal template that has not advanced as quickly as culture has. When you let a man do the work to win you over, you allow him to show you that he, too, recognizes your worth. If a man is not willing to step outside of his comfort zone to get your attention—if he is not capable of picking up the phone to call you, woo you, and earn your trust—then he really is not worth your time, sweet pea.

Date, don't iDate. We're interested in making the actual connection, not the virtual one. We strive to connect viscerally. You want to gaze into the eyes of the one you are interested in, not gaze at your phone when it lights up with one-liner texts from a guy who seems like he could totally live without you.

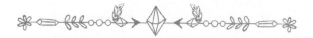

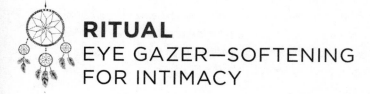

RITUAL
EYE GAZER—SOFTENING FOR INTIMACY

Your body is obedient; it takes your cues and becomes what you spend your time doing. If you are a woman in business and spend all your time shouting orders, being rigid, firm, and "bossy," then you may find that your body is wound up, tight, and tense. When you come home, you want relief from all you've done in the day. You want to be soft. If you want to be taken or consumed by your partner, then you will have to surrender and release the boundaries that get you through the workday. Soften your body to make way for intimacy.

This exercise will help us soften our body and move toward intimacy. As we connect with our partner, we notice the energies as they flow through us. We shift from our thinking heads and become present in our bodies. We allow the other person to see us without pretention or barriers. For those of us in a relationship, we can do this exercise to enhance our relationship with our partner, and those of us who haven't yet partnered can do this exercise with a friend, male or female, to help strengthen our emotional intelligence and ready ourselves for that connection we desire.

Stand with your friend or partner, face-to-face. Gaze at them; see the twinkle in their eyes. Focus on their eyes and their eyes alone. Without touching, engage the breath deep in your belly and breathe nice deep, full breaths while still gazing.

Notice how uncomfortable you become just by looking into the other person. Stay here for 10 minutes and notice what emotions come up for you.

Masculine energy is the organizing principle, and feminine energy is the pleasure principle. After 10 minutes have elapsed, while one person holds the space fixed and steady (masculine), the other person should begin to move rhythmically (feminine), all while still maintaining the gaze. Move freely without touching for two minutes; then switch roles and repeat. Maintain silence and connection. Notice how warm you feel, how your heart is beating. Take a moment to scan your body. Notice the shift in energy created in the space. It's intimate. It's safe, you can relax. Warning: You may need a cool shower after this one!

When Embracing Intimacy Means Embracing Sexuality

When was your last orgasm? If you have to take out the abacus or do long division to figure it out, that needs to change today! We long for connection and are magnetized by attraction and compelled by the urge to merge into oneness. Passion is what connects us to life, and desire is our portal to divine union. Ecstasy is our birthright, and it's the source of all living things. Sex is more than just our single desire as individuals for intimate connection or erotic experiences. It is the most profound expression of the power of creation. The mating drive is one of the most powerful forces in the world. Your sexuality is a mere piece of your primal power and pulsing life force that governs the Universe, and it connects you to that cosmic energy.

How you relate to and operate with that power has an impact on your life. You can repress or restrict it, but it then shows up in other areas of your life. On the other hand, you can embrace it and you can celebrate it. You can learn to consciously open your inner portal to your sexual life force, gain access to divine bliss, and link to your wild glow power, thereby driving yourself farther along this transformative journey.

If you want to have better sex and more satisfying intimate relationships, start with the woman in the mirror—yourself, baby! We embrace our sexuality by learning how our bodies engage in and respond to sex, by creating mental space to allow arousal to stir and knowing when to pull back the reins and push full steam ahead. The more you understand who you are sexually and how you operate, the better you will be in all areas of your life.

Understanding Arousal

What turns you on? No, really think about this. I don't personally need to know, but I want *you* to know and understand your own arousal. Women have an interconnected network of structures that act together to choreograph arousal and orgasm. Sexual arousal is an altered state of consciousness, which means it is a mind-body mode that takes us outside of our ordinary state of awareness into an elevated, trancelike state. (Dreaming, meditation, and even childbirth are other altered states induced by the brain and breath.) Arousal trance is characterized by a deep awareness of bodily sensations, a feeling of warped time and space, and decreased pain perception, resulting in heightened pleasure. Arousal is your guide, and all you have to do is go where it takes you; it taps us into an immediate physical and emotional experience. The capacity for arousal and orgasm is something we are born with. You will have reached full sexual maturity and blossomed into full glow power when you can appropriately use the full spectrum of your core and supplementary powers. Your feminine edge will dominate, and you will operate in full alignment with your authentic self. Being "turned on" in life is tapping into your bliss.

Singing—the Pleasure Principle

When we open up to sing, particularly with songs that have a deep, lower tone, we trigger the use of the vagus nerve, which snakes throughout our body. It innervates the voice box, throat, upper palate, lungs, and parts of the digestive system, as well as the heart. What most people don't know is that the vagus nerve is directly hardwired to the cervix and uterus.

Opening the mouth and chest cavity through slow, meditative deep breathing awakens the vagus nerve and opens a pathway for pleasure. Your energetic singing actually works the muscles in the back of the throat to activate the vagus nerve as well as your sympathetic nervous system. This conducts a feeling of being in a flow state.

A relaxed mouth and jaw while singing may also lead to powerful orgasms. When women emit deep, low sounds that originate from their wombs with their mouths wide open, it can sometimes lead to longer lasting arousal, powerful orgasms, and even female ejaculation—particularly when paired with pelvic pumps or Kegel pulses.

Making moaning and loud sounds while singing creates a powerful release "down and out" of the pelvic floor and genitals, invigorating the depths of the inner sanctum. You might feel this when you are singing full-throated songs. The diaphragm pushes downward on the pelvis. So your singing in the shower is good for you, no matter how you sound.

Your Bliss Button

There are natural ebbs and flows in our sex hormones. We learned about the moon and the menstrual cycle. There are some notable points along your cycle that can enhance your sensuality.

Estrogen peaks with testosterone at the midpoint of the menstrual cycle and makes women more receptive to sex; that estrogen is essential for vaginal lubrication. Testosterone is the main trigger needed to prompt your sexual drive; it naturally rises along with your sexual urges during the second part of your cycle, right before ovulation. This is a great time for outward expression, to go out on a hot date or be social. It's a time when your yang energy is strong and can be leveraged in your favor to embrace intimacy. Progesterone rises in the second part of your cycle, curbing the effects of testosterone on the body. Most women have a decreased interest in sex when progesterone is high in the last part of their menstrual cycle. This is a yin-dominant phase and a good time to turn inward, journal, be alone, meditate, put your rituals into practice, and make clearance.

Haute Sex

In order to get turned on, you have to tune out. Shut off your busy mind so that impulses can rush through the body and ignite the pleasure centers. Multitasking women have an extremely challenging time letting go of their "lists" and surrendering in the bedroom. This boundary prevents the body from completely melting into the throes of passion. I speak to so many women who say, "I had sex because my partner wanted to, but I wasn't really in the mood." It's very important to remember that if you are thinking about your dry cleaning, your to-do list, or your unpaid bills, then you're not allowing the fear and worry center of the brain, the amygdala, to shut off in the way that it needs to for the facilitation of heightened arousal and orgasm. So, what conditions need to be met for you to feel relaxed and in the moment? Is it a hot bath, a glass of champagne, a foot rub, ambiance, or music to set the mood? Turn in and tune out. You owe yourself that experience.

If It Doesn't Feel Good, Don't Do It

I say this all the time. An orgasm can only be triggered if the fear center of the brain has been disengaged. It's really simple: If you're not comfortable, cozy, and content, you're not going to achieve the blastoff of your life. Your body is the arbiter of what is safe. If you are in the bedroom and you are not enjoying sex, stop. It's not a good use of your energy to endure an experience that is not pleasurable. In fact, it's a disrespect to your body. Sex is an act of pleasure—it's a holy experience—and we should be fully present, engaged, and aroused.

When It Feels Good, Do It More

I have met so many women who have not been satisfied sexually, but when they finally find a partner and an arrangement that works for them, they start to feel guilty or make excuses for why it shouldn't work. When you find yourself experiencing a connection, acknowledge it! Don't deny what is happening to you and through you. Getting out of our own way is key. Rather than questioning yourself, stay in the present moment and find all the reasons that it's right!

Self-Love as an Avenue to Greater Intimacy

Embracing your own sexuality goes hand in hand with the concept of reclaiming self-care. Loving your body and understanding how your body works is part and parcel with that. How can we ever truly surrender to our sexual desires and uncover our sexual needs if we don't integrate and celebrate that the body acts as a vessel for them?

Beauty Is an Inside Job

Society constantly makes us feel less than who we are. As a little black girl, I noticed very early on that my skin color was not celebrated in the books I read, on TV, in ad campaigns, or among the dolls I had to choose from. My mother affirmed me with black history and positive imagery and bought me chocolate-skinned Cabbage Patch dolls. Even still, I had to affirm *myself* as I grew up. It's something I do every day. I speak blessings upon myself. I remind myself that I am beautiful. I am not just affirming my appearance, but my existence. I am here both to be and to create beauty.

We are inundated with images of someone else's supposed ideal. As a result, 8 of 10 women do not like what they see when they look in the mirror. We want to appear thinner, taller, and more "beautiful," and we neglect the beauty within. We have to learn how to see beyond the glass. If you're worried about your belly bulge, the freckles on your face, or the kink of your curly locks, know that you are not alone. So many of us objectify ourselves by looking in the mirror and seeing ourselves as a collection of parts and not ourselves as a whole. The mirror does not capture your story and your depth, your world. You are not two-dimensional; you are multifaceted.

The world may not celebrate or acknowledge your beauty, your skin tone, your shape, your size, your hair texture, your teeth, your breast cup, or the circumference of your thighs, but when you look in the mirror, when you strip down to your naked self, what do you see? When you look at your reflection, is it a means of affirmation, checking to see if your outfit looks good, or is it a means for self-criticism? Are you using the mirror to speak blessings on yourself, to gaze upon yourself, and to acknowledge how special you are?

"It's me, and I love me. I've learned to love me. I've been like this my whole life and I embrace me. I love how I look. I am a full woman and I'm strong, and I'm powerful, and I'm beautiful at the same time."

– Serena Williams

RITUAL
FAST FROM YOUR REFLECTION

In an effort to get right with your body and to offset the vanity that we all have, I want you to consider fasting from mirrors. Transform your self-image and focus less on how you look and more on how you want to feel.

How long you fast is up to you, but I want you to commit. Start with a full day. At the beginning of the day, follow your morning routine as usual—washing your face, brushing your teeth, styling your hair. You can go makeup free. Cover your mirrors at home if you feel tempted to look. Ignore the reflective surfaces on the street as you move through your day as well.

For a less intense version of the exercise, you can start the day using the mirror to get ready in the morning and then mirror fast for the remainder of the day, which means no makeup touch-ups outside of refreshing your lipstick, which you can do without looking in the mirror.

Notice what comes up for you emotionally. Write about how this makes you feel.

Do you feel more or less secure in yourself?

How many times are you tempted to look in the mirror?

What's motivating you to look into the mirror?

Are you judging yourself even when you aren't looking in the mirror?

This is a ritual you might incorporate on a regular basis, once a week, or once a month to reset. Perhaps it's part of a dedicated day of glow time. Then we can reaffirm ourselves when we look at our mirrors daily.

Affirming and Reframing Your Reflection

Use lipstick, dry-erase markers, or Post-it notes to place affirmations on the mirrors you use most. Write encouraging mantras and affirmations on your bathroom mirror and place one in your makeup compact so that each time you see yourself, you also see the kind words you've put there to lift you up. When you feel yourself criticizing body parts, reframe those statements: "I hate my thighs" becomes "My thighs are powerful and help support my strong body." It's not about lying to yourself or faking it till you mean it; it's about shattering old patterns of self-destruction. It's about loving your body in the moment and reclaiming your body as sacred one step at a time.

Lather Up with Love

After your shower, while your skin is moist and soft, say your affirmations aloud while massaging a soothing body butter into your skin. Remember, what you put on your skin enters your bloodstream, as the skin is your largest organ. You may be in lust with the coolest new facial serums and body creams, but simple is always best. I recommend a shea butter and coconut-oil blend to keep your skin moisturized and radiant. You can make my recipe at home! Since you use so much on your body, it's most affordable to make it yourself. Remember that a little bit goes a long way when it comes to moisturizing.

YOU ARE NOT THE EXCEPTION. YOU ARE THE EXAMPLE.

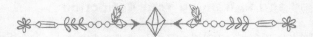

DIY ADORN BODY BUTTER

What you'll need:

    ½ cup shea butter
    ½ cup mango butter
    ½ cup coconut oil
    ½ cup jojoba oil
    Optional: 25 drops of essential oil or flower essence of choice

Directions:

In a double boiler (or glass bowl seated in a pot of water on the stove), combine all ingredients except the essential oil or flower essence.

Bring to medium heat and stir constantly until all ingredients are melted.

Remove from heat and add the essential oil or flower essence.

Refrigerate for 1 hour or until the mixture starts to harden.

Use a hand mixer to whip for 10 minutes until fluffy.

Return to fridge for 10 to 15 minutes to set.

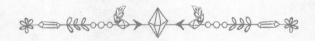

RITUAL
HAMMAM AT HOME

One of the most decadent and nurturing experiences for the body is the Hammam ritual, where exfoliation and deep cleansing work to purify the body. This is a head-to-toe ritual that leaves skin as smooth as silk. The Hammam is likely the oldest surviving bath tradition in the world. The ruins of the oldest known Islamic Hammam in Morocco dates back to the late eighth century. Traditionally speaking, the Hammam was more than just a bath house; it was also a place where people gathered for glow time.

Hammam treatments include many beneficial components, from warm, steamy, circulating air to vigorous exfoliation to sensual or therapeutic massages. The results are glowing skin and rejuvenation.

Create your own Hammam at home. Light some candles, turn on your playlist, and start your steamy ceremony.

Blow off steam. Create your own sauna-like atmosphere at home by letting the hot shower run until the room becomes steamy and warm. You can place five drops of eucalyptus or rosemary essential oil in a diffuser to infuse the air with a cleansing aromatic scent.

Soap it up. Moroccan black soap is used in traditional Hammams to pull impurities from the pores. Lather with a rich creamy soap. If you can't find black soap, olive oil or Shea butter-based soap will do.

Exfoliate. The Hammam is best known for exfoliation. Sloughing off dead skin cells is achieved with a glove called a kessa. Massage the skin in circular motions to help bring new skin to the surface. You can also use a body scrub here instead of the glove.

Purify. This is an optional step in the process. Massage a thin layer of body mud into the skin for purifying and revitalizing effects. Let the mask sit on the skin for two minutes, then rinse off.

Moisturize and massage. After rinsing, your supple skin will be ready for moisturizing. Apply argan oil directly to your exfoliated skin after stepping from the steamy shower. Argan oil is lightweight and absorbs easily into the skin. Blend pure argan oil with a sensual flower essence like orange blossom or rose for an inviting and soothing body massage.

Hydrate. Remember to stay hydrated during this process. Keep a pitcher of water or a water bottle in the bathroom and sip frequently while steaming and throughout your home Hammam ritual.

Putting On Your Power Suit

Like most girls growing up in the '80s, I had an obsession with Wonder Woman. Sure, Wonder Woman *could have* worn civilian clothes when she moved about town fighting evil, but instead, she wore a glittery, skin-tight halter leotard, a flashy belt accentuating her cinched waistline, knee-high kinky boots, her signature red cape, and a matching headband holding her Farrah Fawcett hairdo perfectly in place. She evoked a feeling of power with her fierce femininity and strength. She owned her glow.

What's your Wonder Woman look? I don't mean your costume. I mean, what makes you feel powerful when you have it on? The clothes we adorn ourselves with should be both a statement of power to the outside world and a reaffirmation to ourselves of our own strength and limitless potential.

What we wear isn't just a statement about how we think of ourselves. It can actually affect how we feel about ourselves. Studies have shown that such a phenomenon exists. Hajo Adam and Adam Galinsky, cognitive psychologists at Northwestern University, conducted a study that found that the clothing we wear affects our psychological state as well as our performance level. In the study, they dressed people in what they believed to be a doctor's coat and others in what they believed to be a painter's coat and measured the psychological changes. Each group was wearing the same white coat. Those who thought the coat was a doctor's showed improved ability to pay attention and to focus on detail. Those who thought their coats were for painters did not show any differences. Also, those who wore the "doctor's" coats performed better on a test than those who wore regular clothing. Adam and Galinsky coined the term *enclothed cognition*, which captures the influence that clothes have on the psychological processes of the person wearing them.

So, knowing how influential the clothing we wear is to our psychological state and the quality of our performance, what should we wear? How can we use clothing to induce desirable psychological states and enhance task-related performance? Every superheroine has to have her own version of the cape and leotards and a whole lot of spandex. What's your power look? What is your strongest silhouette? How do you speak with your clothing? What does it say about you? Are you dressing for the job and money you deserve? Are you forgetting to add your foxy femme touch? If you are what you wear, how can you dress to your advantage?

To enhance your creative power and honor your feminine edge, dress in clothes that evoke that particular feeling you want to transmit, both to yourself and to the outside world. Reframe "getting dressed" to "adorning yourself," and suddenly the moments you spend preparing yourself for the day are charged with ritual quality. What you wear and how you wear it are a healthy and artistic form of self-expression. From scarves and ascots to tribal bibs, there are many ways to show the world who you are and what you value. What's important is not to be overwhelmed by your options.

Get Out of the Rut

You know you're in a rut with your personal style when you open the closet and find not a single thing to wear. We constantly grow and evolve, and so should our wardrobes. When my son was three, he decided he wanted to pick out his own clothes. "Clothes give you power," he said. Wise words. We want to wear what makes us feel most potent.

Recognize when you feel like you need a fashion overhaul. It's a sign that you need to augment your power. Identifying those definitive wardrobe pieces might go a long way toward *helping* define your look. But let's get out of the rut first and *then* find our signature look.

It's a great exercise to regularly clear out your closet. I recommend doing so twice a year. Purging your closets will not only help you see more effectively what it is you have to wear, but it will also help you acquire new finds more effectively. You will find pieces you forgot about, things you may have outgrown—physically and in personality—things you hope to wear again, and things you wish you'd never bought. And then there are pieces that transcend time, that are definitive wardrobe pieces that you should hold on to. The things that you don't love, you give up. The things that don't make you feel sexy, smart, and powerful, you give up. If you have trouble discerning what to keep and what to toss, invite a trusted friend or two who can help you purge your closet. Make two piles: "love it" and "leave it." Whatever goes into the "leave it" pile is on its way to help someone else on their journey. It's already taken you as far as it can; you're off to bigger and better things now.

Explore Your Signature Look

If you've ever gone through six outfits, ending up with a pile of clothes on the floor as you're trying to make your exit to go somewhere, then you know from experience that it can be challenging to nail your best look. Often, we unnecessarily complicate our style because we aren't sure of who we wish to portray to the world. But zeroing in on your personal style does not have to be a daunting process, and it doesn't have to cost a fortune, either. Let's walk through some basic principles for simplifying style and making it personal so that it's appropriate for the boardroom, the bar, or a ball.

What types of looks are you drawn to in others?

What is your current go-to outfit, and what do you love about it?

Do you consider yourself more modest, or do you like to push boundaries?

What three adjectives would you use to describe the spirit that you want your clothes to help you embody? (fiery, serious, warm, and so on)

What accessories do you gravitate toward?

What colors inspire you?

Are there particular brands that you love?

What celebrity or influencer style speaks to you most?

Which parts of your body do you want to accentuate?

When you ask these questions first, you can target a signature look that meets all the above criteria. You can incorporate the staples in your closet that feel good and help you present your strongest and most confident self to the world. Take the guesswork out of choosing an outfit every morning and instead give yourself room to play with *embellishing* that standard look in fun and exciting ways.

Ways to Play with Your Style

Having an edge is all about reaching beyond the lines of the status quo and establishing your own unique identity. Your personal style reflects so much about who you are. It's not defined just by the type of clothes you like to wear; it's also influenced by your friends, your career path, where you live, your hobbies, and your aspirations. You should dress for the dreams you have. On your quest to defining your signature look, try experimenting with these different elements of style until you find what works for you!

Proportion

A shift dress, a halter, a skinny pant. Say our signature look is the little black dress. A little black shift dress make us feel confident in the boardroom, but we might want to try it in a halter style for a night out on the town. It depends on what you want to accentuate. Play with the silhouettes and lines in your look.

Pattern

Pattern is about being bold, taking risks, showing character, having a larger-than-life personality, and displaying confidence. If you're shy, patterns can help you step outside of your comfort zone. Not ready for bold patterns in your blouses, dresses, or slacks? You can take a classic look you're comfortable with and use accessories—scarves, shoes, bags—to bump up the boldness.

Texture

Not everything you wear has to be the same texture. Texture connotes depth, personality, and maturity. Taking a woven or knit blouse and pairing it with a pleated skirt brings dimension to your look.

Color

The colors we wear can have a powerful effect on our energy. Wear white to calm your energy field, blue to nurture your spirit, yellow to energize your aura, red to gather your force, and red and black when you need a little spice and mischief in your life.

Contrast

Color blocking shows your confidence and can accentuate certain features, pulling a look together. Playing with lights and darks can connote that you're serious and makes a powerful statement in the boardroom.

Synergy

Embrace the cohesive look. Sometimes we want to wear a few amazing pieces all at once but they don't work together. You can keep your look balanced by adding *one* statement piece of jewelry and forgo the piling on of too many pieces.

Don't Be Daunted by Trends

Personal style is not driven by, but accented by, trends. Since trends change by the season, you will grow exhausted trying to keep up with what "should" be in your wardrobe. Rather than changing your style every season, just take what excites you and fold it into what your wardrobe already consists of. You always want to feel comfortable in your own skin and in your own closet. If a look doesn't flatter you, don't wear it. Not every trend is right for every person, and if it doesn't make you feel your strongest, then it's not worth it.

Before you buy a trendy piece, make sure there are at least three different outfits you see yourself wearing it with from items that are already part of your closet. If you think you will live in this new piece, it likely complements your style. If you're having a hard time imagining how or when you might incorporate it, it's probably not meant to be. When in doubt about a trend you're drawn to, accessorize with bags, shoes, tights, a wallet, or statement jewelry. Instead of a head-to-toe lace jumpsuit, how about a camisole with a delicate touch of lace at the décolletage, nodding to the trend without bowing to it?

Put the "Chic" Back in "Cozy Chic"

Are you the type who wishes she could wear yoga pants to the office, to the gym, and on a date? I have a secret to share: You can look put together and still be comfortable. You don't need to wear stilettos or a corset to the supermarket to flaunt your personal style. There is definitely a happy medium. When you coordinate punches of color, even when wearing your gym clothes, you'll look amazing. You can dress a seemingly more casual, less restricting outfit up with a scarf or statement necklace. Maxi shirts and dresses are a comfy alternative to those yoga pants you have been wearing all day long.

If you *must* wear leggings, try embellished ones. For example, American Apparel makes a faux-leather pant that looks more expensive and stylish than any pair of leather pants I've seen, and you can throw them in the wash! Accent your leggings with a nice pair of boots or booties, creating a comfortable and sleek silhouette.

It's only acceptable to walk around in sweats if you're a performance athlete or when you're sick with the flu. If you're neither, toss the sweats. I'm all for hoodies, but ditch the sweatpants. There are better ways to be comfortable and still be your best self!

Your Underwear: The First Layer of Your Power Suit

I love to wear beautiful undergarments, and I do it for myself, not for my partner. When we adorn ourselves with nice-fitting and flattering clothing, it makes us feel good about ourselves. When we do it with our underwear, it's a little way of honoring our sacred female anatomy. We have to upgrade our panty sets to reflect who we are and how we want to feel. Ladies, you're worth it. Clear out the old stuff and granny panties that you don't love and make space for your superheroine-power panties. Don't just pull out the "good stuff" for your partner or when you have a hot date. Every day you get dressed is a mini celebration of how good it is to be *you*! Wear panties that make you feel powerful! Shop for undergarments that you would feel proud of if someone saw you in them. You have the sunshine between your thighs. Dress like it!

Wearing beautiful undergarments doesn't need to be constricting. I recently visited the Negative Underwear showroom, where I talked to the founders about their beautiful, well-edited line of functional undergarments and tanks. I tried on some very comfortable bras that felt like I wasn't wearing anything at all. And they were beautiful! Marissa Vosper, a cofounder of the brand, says,

> We started Negative because we saw a real gap in the market. For women who cared quite a bit about the clothes we wore, our underwear was usually an afterthought . . . We wanted to make better underwear for every day—uncomplicated, considered, and minimal. A line that was as comfortable and functional as it was beautiful and cool.

So, go online and shop the many retailers that have beautiful collections you can invest in. Ditch the granny panties. Hello, Agent Provocateur and Kiki de Montparnasse!

A Note about the Best Underwear for Your Cycle

When your cycle comes, you want to put your cherished lace thongs aside and wear something that provides coverage and support but still makes you feel amazing. Companies like THINX are reimagining menstruation for women around the world. THINX not only provides solutions for women having their periods, they take the shame out of monthly menses. The pieces are handcrafted by women in Sri Lanka, and they also have a social mission to support young women in Uganda who have limited access to feminine-hygiene products and, as a result, aren't able to attend school. Also, be sure that any tampons or pads you use are made with organic cotton. Being empowered down to your panties is just another step toward owning your glow.

RITUAL
UNCLOAKING THE GODDESS

When you were little and believed in superheroines, you dressed up like them and imagined that you were Superwoman, She-Ra, Xena the Warrior Princess, Storm, Jem—the list goes on. So now as adults, we need to ignite within ourselves the aspects of the superheroine that speaks to our soul. It's like putting on a cape and playing make-believe. Wear that goddess energy on your shirtsleeve and drape yourself in your power.

Explore folklore from around the globe to discover which goddess feels most aligned with your energy. You could look at embodying aspects of the Triple Goddess. It could even be a historical, archetypal "goddess" like Cleopatra or a modern-day, living goddess embodied like Beyoncé. I like to look to folklore because there are archetypes associated with the different goddess energies, and you can pick and choose what aspects you want to evoke, ignite within, and embody.

When you wake up in the morning, take a few minutes to ground yourself in how you want to feel, who you want to be this day. What goddess or superheroine attributes do you want to embody today? When you've identified the feeling you want to embody, mindfully walk over to your closet and pick out the garments that best reflect the feelings and attributes you want to express. Adorn yourself in accessories that also speak to the feeling you are cultivating, including necklaces, bracelets, earrings, rings, belts, hats, or scarves. Be mindful of how you walk cloaked as a living goddess. What attitude and frame of mind do you need to lean into to unleash the energy of the goddess within?

Notice what happens when you walk in the vibration and energy of the goddess. How do you perceive yourself? What will be your attributes today? How will you finesse each interaction? When you undress, take a moment to reflect upon how you felt in that particular outfit.

You can do this ritual before going out on a hot date, job interview, a business meeting, or any special occasion.

Did you not find exactly what you were looking for? Go through your closet and edit for the best pieces and go shopping for pieces that evoke the feeling and mood you want to express through your wardrobe. It could be as simple as an accessory like a scarf or hat, hairpins or stockings, or full-on pieces for your closet.

glow tips for
Amplifying Your Style

Do Goodwill. Any clothes you decide to part with can help another person in need. Consider donating your gently used clothes and shoes to Goodwill and allowing someone else to put your once-treasured pieces to good use. When you clear your closet of old clothes, you make space for new pieces, and you can actually see what amazing looks you have on hand.

Get styled! If you have a stylist in your life or a friend who has incredible style, enlist that person to help you with building up your wardrobe. It's not a show of weakness to have someone who knows you well pick out clothes that are a reflection of who you are at your best. It's often easier with someone who can help you navigate the brands, the stores, and the trends. Style icon June Ambrose is a friend whom I call whenever I get stuck. When I had to attend a polo tournament, June texted me style-inspiration images so that when I went shopping, I knew what I was looking for.

Get inspired. Bookmark your favorite sites and blogs for style and fashion and regularly visit them. Give yourself a limit to how long you'll spend surfing for inspiration, and see what you find. Don't just look in the obvious places. Websites like One King's Lane are like porn for interior decorators, but they have one-of-a-kind accessory finds, too. And I've found wallpaper prints that have inspired me to have a pair of classic pumps finished in a textile pattern I found from traditional Indian sari scraps.

Mix high and low. Got a $19 find from Forever 21 that you want to merchandise up with an amazing ready-to-wear piece? Perfectly acceptable! Mixing high and low fashions is key to style versatility and saving on your wardrobe. Try raiding your local consignment, thrift, and resale stores for cool designer pieces that can bring your closet history, heritage, and character. You might stumble upon a vintage goldmine and be the only one who knows about it! Don't be pressured to mimic the expensive designer looks you see in magazines. No one needs a look straight off the catwalk unless she's headed straight to the red carpet. Mixing it up will cement your style credentials rather than undermine them.

Know (and love) your body type. Find out what works for your body type and embrace the styles that work for your shape. Some women are curvy, and others have straight figures. Some are pear shaped, and some have long torsos. There are different ways to accent and emphasize your body shape so that you always feel like you're celebrating your assets!

Embrace color. For some reason, in New York, it's all-black everything, all year round. By winter, most items are gray or shades of black. But don't retreat into the dullness of the black outfit; punch it up with color. Layer with a teal-green sweater, add a little pop with a colorful wool scarf, or sport a fun shoe. Look to alternative shades to the primary color block to bring some bold tones into the mix. Even a touch of color on your lips will boost your mood and brighten your skin tone. Like style maven and TV personality Tai Beauchamp says, "Never leave the house without red lipstick."

Be you! I can't reiterate this enough. You want to express what is within, and your signature design looks should complement and accent your existing style. An understanding of who you are and who you want to become when you are dressed is important. Your wardrobe should work to your benefit. You're wearing the clothes—the clothes are not wearing you!

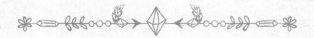

All the steps in this chapter are here to help us along the journey to owning our glow. From sexuality to setting boundaries, menstrual cycles to self-care, self-acceptance to personal style, all these things advance us on our journey toward creatively living our purpose-driven life.

"I believe that fashion, style and dressing are really great ways for women to express and interact with their creativity, and that's an empowering thing."

- Zac Posen,
fashion designer

glow guidance

"When someone finds the right mentor, it is obvious. Chasing or forcing that connection rarely works."

~ SHERYL SANDBERG, *LEAN IN*

Glow guidance is unwavering support given through mentorship, friendship, and good deeds. You should consider your glow guides your soul's board of directors. They are invested in your personal growth and success and have unique skills to offer you. Identify your cheerleaders early on, confide in your glow guides, and allow them to shine light on your experiences. And as you become more comfortable in your glow, begin to shine that light on others.

In this chapter, we will explore criteria for choosing glow guides, discuss how best to incorporate glow guidance into our lives—both as a mentee and a mentor—talk about building friendships grounded in accountability and trust, and think about how else we might embody our glow power in the way we give to those around us. We are blessed. It is important to pay it forward and support up-and-comers and those whom we don't know personally but who might benefit from our light. Find a meaningful way to give back that strikes a chord with you, whether that's teaching yoga to teen girls, taking one day of your vacation and spending it with people in need, or supporting a local environmental cause. This feels especially good when you are in need of the support you are offering. For instance, if you feel lonely or nostalgic about family, visit residents at a local nursing home.

How to Find Your Mentor

A mentor's job is to be a trusted advisor who models positive behavior and is tuned in to your needs, offering advice and support to launch you to the next level. Busy people want to invest in others they believe will yield results. Mentors are cheerleaders; they are there for support, troubleshooting, and confidence building. They are not meant to map out your journey and do the work for you. They are there to enhance your experience, to inspire, to ask you the challenging questions, and be glowing images of aspiration.

I've had several informal mentors over the years, mostly people who were in completely different careers but saw my spirit and potential and decided to invest in me. It wasn't necessary for them to be in my particular professional field. The idea is not to look at *what* people do, but how they do it. It's about finding people whose energy and drive are admirable and inspirational. It's about aligning yourself with a mentor who will guide you to achieving your goals with grace and fortitude—and believe in you.

For those looking for mentors within your industries, find them among the people you know who are 10 steps ahead of you, doing what you want to do, in the way you envision yourself doing it.

You can find great mentors within the circle of people you're already interacting or working with now. They need to be people to whom you have already demonstrated your potential—who have seen how you think, move, and communicate and who understand the contributions you're making or have already made. They have to like, trust, and believe in you and feel you'll put all their input and advice to great use.

Connect with new people whom you know *you* can help in return and who will find it a mutually rewarding and beneficial experience. It needs to feel good to support you. Are you somebody you yourself would like to mentor? Are you open, flexible, resilient, respectful, and unstoppable? Are you eager to learn and committed to pivoting in your interactions so you can become your best self and have more success, rewards, and happiness?

Harness the Networking Experience

Debra Lee, CEO of BET Networks, is someone I consider a mentor. Our relationship started when I became her private yoga instructor, but it evolved to where she became invested in my success after getting to know me. She includes me in events and opportunities, and we share good conversation. I make suggestions and support her where my strengths lie. I give.

Networking is about identifying people we'd love to connect with who excite and inspire us, reaching out to offer *our* help through our connections and know-how, and keeping the giving coming. Acquiring a mentor should be about taking your time and watering the garden for the relationship to flourish. *Then* we get.

Strangers Do Not Mentors Make

Asking a complete stranger whom you follow or admire from afar is not the best way to acquire a mentor. If people have no relationship with you, they don't know how you operate or what kind of time commitment is required to help you. In fact, if you build up the courage to ask for their support, you will likely find that they decline your request.

People in the media and the public eye who have become highly visible successes are frequently forced to say no to mentoring requests from strangers, because their time is already spoken for and they're already inundated with similar requests. If you think you're inspired by a certain person, what about the thousands of other folks who are inspired right along with you? That isn't to say that you can't watch their steps, read their interviews, and glean wisdom from their actions. By all means, learn everything you can from those who are getting theirs and doing it gracefully. But don't expect them to fill the role of mentor. If you *do* have the opportunity to speak or connect with such a person, ask a poignant question instead. Allow them to gift you with their wisdom and be grateful to the Universe for sending them at the right time.

If you *haven't* yet met someone, don't ask for mentorship, but do follow their work and be supportive. If you have social-media accounts, use that space to *give*. Tweet out people's posts, comment in a positive way on their blogs, share their updates, start a discussion on Facebook or LinkedIn that draws on their post, refer new clients or business to them. Offer your unique voice, perspective, experience, and resources to further the action and conversation that these influencers have sparked inside of you. This is a great way for them to see that you are genuinely interested in them and not just what they can offer you. Understand that even though you may not be at the same stage in life or have comparable experience, you may still be of great service to them. Find a way to serve, without stepping on their toes. If you see an area of growing edge where they could use help or support in an area where you have strengths, share your idea with them. That may just lead you to an acquaintanceship.

glow tips for

Attracting and Honoring Empowered Mentorship

Be all that you can be. While this sounds obvious, it is the most important thing you can do to get noticed. Be great at what you do.

Seek more responsibility in your position. Be sure to have specific ideas for how you can contribute in deeper, more expansive ways. Be creative and think outside the box.

Don't be shy. Participate in all meetings, even "optional" ones. Volunteer to represent your team on important department- or enterprise-level initiatives. Share your ideas. Prepare ahead of time so that you can meaningfully advance the discussion.

Promote the success of those around you. Your generosity and openness are critical to your personal success.

Build your network. Reach out to community groups both within your company and outside your line of business, including communities like Levo League, Rising Tide Society, Career Contessa, General Assembly, OKREAL, and Create & Cultivate. Learn what they do and how you can help them succeed and what you can learn and bring to the conversation.

Ask yourself what you want in a mentor. Is it an expert who can help with a specific challenge—asking for a raise, transitioning to a new career, improving your image and personal style? Do you want someone inside your workplace, someone who has the inside track to be an advocate for your project or promotion? Or do you want someone outside the workspace who can act as a more general sounding board and big-picture guide?

Put yourself in a potential mentor's shoes. If the tables were turned, what would you want to see from this individual asking for help? If you were inundated with requests for guidance every day, what type of person would you choose to assist, and why? Become the person that others would love to support and nurture.

The fortune is in the follow-up. Don't let your contacts lie dormant. A business card should be more than a piece of paper whose life cycle ends in the bottom of your purse. It's a calling card to opportunity, a seed of potential for connection. Take five business cards in your possession right now and reach out to those contacts. How can you deepen those relationships?

Accelerator programs. Accelerator programs are fixed-term, cohort-based, and include mentorship and educational opportunities under the guidance of one or more mentors and advisors. They range in intensity and can be free of charge or can cost the mentee. If you are really keen on working with a particular person, ask if he or she offers coaching or an accelerator program.

Bring out the fun in mentoring you! When making your ask, consider how it comes across. You don't want to make it sound like work. Exude excitement and smiles. Mentorship is an invigorating opportunity for both parties, and when done properly, it often blooms into a friendship. Once you've acquired a mentor, find ways to meet regularly with purpose, even without an urgent agenda. Nurture the relationship year-round. Send nice handwritten notes or a gift. Let them know they are appreciated for their friendship as much as for their help.

Show your mentor how to help you. Even after some-one's decided they want to help you, most won't know where to start. Make a specific request when you want someone to speak up on your behalf. Don't flounder or beat around the bush. They'll appreciate the guidance and perspective.

Honor your mentor. Show your gratitude for the invalu-able support. Where it's possible to reciprocate, become a source of service. Do you have some information and support that may be valuable to your mentor? Share it. When you have tickets to an event someone might enjoy, invite them. Don't just think about mentors when you need something. Keep them at the front of your mind, and you will distinguish yourself and remain at the top of their list as well.

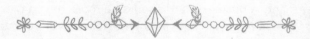

The answers to many of your questions aren't as far away as they seem. They're right inside of you. Those who are closest to the problem are closest to the solution. Understand that you have much more to offer than you realize. You may need mentoring in some areas of your life, and in others you may already be a mentor yourself. Stepping into the shoes of your inner mentor will help you spread the glow and fuel your glow power by boosting your self-confidence and self-worth through helping others.

RESOURCEFULNESS IS NOT JUST ABOUT TURNING IDEAS INTO OPPORTUNITIES. IT'S ABOUT TURNING INFLUENCE INTO LEVERAGE.

The Push

Somebody pushed me in this direction and helped me get to where I am. There was a time when I didn't fully believe in myself. Thankfully, there were people who saw far beyond what I could see for myself. My friend and florist Saundra Parks was one of those people whose encouragement traveled with me a long way while I built my self-confidence in business. Saundra was so helpful in spreading the word about my work even when I wasn't fully ready to step into my power. You don't have to be an influencer, a person who's well connected, impactful, sought after, and in-the-know, to have been an influential person in someone else's life. There are people who have no idea that I admired them and watched their trajectory from afar, but their perseverance gave me juice to push through the barriers. In the same way, there are likely people in your life who probably have no idea how influential they were along your journey. They may not know that they taught you something invaluable, that they pushed you in the direction of growth.

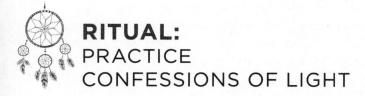

RITUAL:
PRACTICE
CONFESSIONS OF LIGHT

Confessions of light are an opportunity to speak about inspiration and acknowledge people who have made a beauty mark on your life. As you prepare to use your own power and influence to the benefit of others, you want to be sure to reach out to those who helped push *you* along the way.

This practice allows us to practice gratitude and appreciate how blessed we are when faced with the biggest challenges and smallest challenges. It also makes our army of angels feel appreciated and connected to their purpose in service. This is a weekly practice for me, but you can do it daily or however often it feels best.

Make a short list of people to whom you want to confess.

Take a moment to call or text or voice memo those people and confess to them what you are grateful for. If you can devote more than a few minutes, consider confessing with a post on Instagram or writing a greeting card.

Take out your journal and soul-scribe:

Make a list of people who've pushed you.

How have they been most influential in your life?

Who in your universe needs a push?

How will you use your influence to push others?

Who will you confess your appreciation to?

How to Optimize Time with Your Mentees

Most mentors have more than one mentee and are strapped for time. I have mentees from all industries and backgrounds. I am always thinking of new ways to serve that don't take up more of my time than I can afford to give. I am interested in investing time in the right relationships, not wasting time. If you are interested in mentoring or maximizing your relationships and service to your current mentees, here are some great ways to connect, engage, and inspire those who look up to you and value your support.

Walk and talk. Take mentees on a walk. It's easy to check in and give advice that way. If you don't get lots of exercise, this could be a way to keep your mind sharp, get fresh air, and visit with your mentees at the same time. Have them meet you at your office, slide on a pair of sneakers, and go for a speed walk while catching up.

Go out to lunch. Hold one lunch a month, or every quarter, and invite mentees to meet you and each other and ask questions. Whoever can make it, comes. Set an agenda for questions—one burning question per mentee. That way everyone leaves with value directly relatable to their personal dilemma or challenge.

Participate in conferences. Go to places where you can offer your mentoring in a contained and effective context. I spoke at the Create & Cultivate Conference in Chicago and served as a mentor in an organized mentor session where 5 tables of 10 women each sat with me and shared their goals, dreams, and challenges, and I offered keen advice and action steps. In two hours, I was able to directly touch the lives of 50 women and their businesses. I even stayed in contact with a few and offer my support when needed.

Broker a mentor. You're not always going to be able to serve everyone who comes to you, and those looking for mentors should know that the people they admire and aspire to be like are very busy and in demand. In some cases, the person seeking your help may not be ready for you and vice versa; perhaps you can connect them with someone better suited to their needs instead. If you don't have the capacity to mentor but would like to support those approaching you, take 20 to 30 minutes for a call to get to know the potential mentee, then cruise through your contact list and see if you can help her find the right fit.

Frequency and Location of Mentorship

How often you connect with your mentees really depends on how much time you can allocate and the task at hand. Lots of mentors use Google Hangouts, phone calls, or Skype to have check-ins with their mentees since it can be a challenge to meet in person. You can also mentor people in other parts of the world if you use these options. You can also take on a larger group and host Facebook live or Instagram live sessions where you answer specific questions and offer advice that touches more than one person. Be specific and honest about your bandwidth from the beginning to manage expectations of your involvement. Healthy boundaries are a must. You should set hours and a schedule so you can have a momentum and accountability structure and not receive phone calls and texts from your mentee(s) constantly.

How to Listen to Your Mentee with Compassion

Listening is not about being polite; it is about witnessing another and being witnessed. Here are some best practices.

Be present. Offer the speaker your full and undivided attention. Put your cell phone away. Look into their eyes. I always say to my son, "When you are in conversation, see the person's eye color." Be that attentive with your gaze and really give your listening ear.

Show interest. Be generous with the space, lean in, and nod your head in affirmation. Ask questions that help the story unfold. Encourage the speaker. Use your facial expression to emote and show your engagement.

Create a safe zone. Hold space for compassion so the person speaking feels safe enough to share. Touch transmits intention; reach out and hold a hand. Your energy transmits a force field that precedes you. Acknowledge the person for their sharing and vulnerability. Release judgment.

Don't interrupt. Listen to every word intently without interrupting. This can be a challenge. Don't focus on how you want to respond, but stay with the speaker. You can pose clarifying questions or otherwise move the conversation forward after the other person has finished his or her thought.

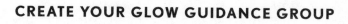

CREATE YOUR GLOW GUIDANCE GROUP

Sometimes instead of mentoring, what we need is to surround ourselves with friends and colleagues who will hold us and for whom we can provide that same service. Find people who are in the same space in development and those who are farther along as well.

Gather the group. Create a group of 3 to 10 people (the smaller, the better) who can come together, ignite each other to play big, and hold each other accountable.

Check in. Accountability is set by regular check-ins. Create an agenda, set goals, and check in on progress weekly. Lift anyone who may be feeling challenged and use this group as a training ground for testing new ideas and getting support.

Use the sister system. Find a buddy in the group and partner up for more targeted support. Perhaps switch partners along the way to see if your perspectives change. This way, you each get more out of working with a new energy.

Take it seriously. When you show up mentally and emotionally to participate, magic happens. Be regular with your attendance. When one person doesn't show up, it weakens the collective.

THERE IS A DIFFERENCE BETWEEN SEEKING INSIGHT AND SEEKING ANSWERS. WHAT ARE YOU SEEKING?

Glow Guidance Reflections

Am I willing to experience discomfort and move beyond my previous limitations to grow and evolve, as guided by those who believe in me?

Am I willing to trust my glow guides and shift my behaviors to support the activation of new behaviors that are aligned with my goals?

Am I willing to embrace the wisdom of a mentor, knowing that it will change the course of my journey?

Are there parts of me that resist creating a new foundation?

Am I willing to dive in and do the work and emerge a better person?

Am I willing to share that guidance and wisdom with those who come after me?

"The secret to elevating your career
is knowing that you are the most powerful
change agent in your own journey."

- Tiffany Dufu

glow grazing

> *"No matter how developed you are in any other area of your life, no matter what you say you believe, no matter how sophisticated or enlightened you think you are, how you eat tells all."*
>
> ~ GENEEN ROTH, *WOMEN FOOD AND GOD*

Have you ever had a bad hair day, where your hair just wasn't right and you didn't feel as beautiful? What about a bad food day, where you ate crappy food and your mood suffered? Maybe you skipped a week at the gym because of stress at work or binged on fast food while on a road trip, or went on a Twizzler and Ben and Jerry's diet because you just broke up? I always say, "You can't save the world if you're eating Skittles," and I really mean it. These fringe foods send your body into a state of chaos. Your kidneys, pancreas, and liver have to work in overdrive to digest these processed foods, and guess what, they get stored in the body as fat! A diet of healthy whole foods is needed to get the abundant nutrition to boost your glow power!

Food carries important information to us about the ambient landscape in which we live. The food you eat becomes your blood, your thoughts, and your actions. Therefore we need to consider the energy of the foods we are putting into our body. The foods that many of us eat, loaded with chemical additives, have effects on our brains and cause hormonal disruption, foggy thinking, weight gain, and dehydration.

Over the years, I've studied food, done nutrition course work, and learned a lot about how my body responds to what I eat. I personally feel my very best on a vegan diet with lots of raw foods in the summertime and green juice and blended smoothies year-round. This is a diet I maintained throughout my pregnancy and that I encourage through any major life transition or period of personal growth. I consider this not only basic good nutrition, but powerful medicine, too. I adhere to a plant-based/vegan diet of leafy greens, whole grains, nuts, seeds, beans, low-glycemic fruits, and high-quality oils and fats. Do you have to be vegan to benefit from this book? Absolutely not! But if you incorporate even a small fraction of the dietary advice you find here, you'll start feeling and looking more radiant and accessing parts of your creative self you never thought possible. You will think more clearly and be more receptive to your creative energy and ideas.

I grew up in Oakland, California. And although it was, for the most part, an urban environment, I was still surrounded by lush hills, gardens, and all the bounty they provided. I knew exactly what route to take home from school so that I could pass the blackberry bushes in the late spring. I would walk with my friends, squeezing the delicate berries off the bushes, our fingers covered in juice that would stain the white Peter Pan collars of our school uniforms—which my mother wasn't happy about. My cousin and I knew just when to pick the sour plums from our neighbor's tree so they had the perfect sour crunchiness. My grandmother introduced me to pickling when I was three! And later, I would pick the growing garden vegetables that she turned into soup. Voilà—magic.

And it wasn't just at Grandma's house. When I was young, I was surrounded by urban gardening. People grew herbs on the window-sill or along the side of the house. Gorgeous fruits and vegetables had a peculiar way of sprouting up in the ever-forgiving soil that's native to my hometown. I didn't realize the extent to which my upbringing had fostered my connection to food until I moved to New York City. It was in New York that the absence of any environmental connection would spark a desire within me to really embrace farm-to-fork.

Knowing and caring about where our food comes from, how it was grown, and how and where it was prepared creates a state of mindfulness about what we eat, a reverence for the environment, and a respect for the people who work to supply our food. What we put in our bodies is an essential part of radical self-care and will help us embody the principles of owning our glow, keeping us open to the whispers of our GPS, allowing us to be our most creative and productive selves.

Do you want to feel great, look great, and boost your mood, energy, and libido? Then I encourage you to be more mindful of the foods you eat. What's really on your plate? Recognize your body as a temple and ask yourself if you are honoring it each time you sit down to eat. This doesn't mean you can't indulge and have treats; it just means you shouldn't have pizza every day!

The medicinal value of food has been acknowledged for thousands of years. Our ancestors were connected to the land, and there was a symbiotic relationship among the land, the surrounding plants and animals, and our bodies. Modern scientific research has gone on to prove that our ancestors were on to something, showing hundreds of beneficial nutrients in the foods that we eat.

We now know that incorporating phytonutrients found in plant foods into our diet helps us boost our immune systems. It's for this reason that I encourage you to explore **glow foods**—superfoods packed with antioxidants, minerals, and powerful nutrients that help combat inflammation, balance the hormonal system, keep insulin levels low, and promote healthy weight management. When you start eating this way, your skin, nails, and hair will shimmer, and you will think more clearly.

When your body is in a state of equilibrium, you are more likely to put *you* first, because you already feel good and want to maintain that feeling. Addressing our diet is a *step* on our progressive journey to owning our glow. When we feel good, we make better choices, and when we eat in a way that satisfies our needs, we keep the energetic channels clear. Food is here to fortify us along the journey.

Experimenting with Glow Foods

It's easy to slide into the same habits and eat the same things over and over. Even if it's your favorite avocado toast, there is such a thing as too much of a good thing. Expand your world by opening yourself to the possibilities of different foods. Buy an ingredient you've never used before and integrate it into a meal.

Don't just try new things; try new things with the purpose of examining how they affect your body. Look at your body as if it were a laboratory and consciously experiment with your foods. Do a breakfast trial, for instance, at the beginning of the new season to see which foods resonate best in the cold or warm months and help jump-start your day. When you experiment with a new food, record three things: how it tasted to you, how you felt before you ate it, and how you felt 30 minutes after you ate it.

The body speaks and expresses itself through sensation. If you eat something and it causes you gas, that's the body telling you something. We want to choose foods that work harmoniously with our bodies and integrate the information we get from food.

What you eat and when you eat have an effect on your mood. I know I need to have breakfast in the morning, because I will have foggy thinking and be in a snappy mood if I don't eat well. Eat the foods that you've learned work for you personally, that help sustain your mood, energy level, and libido.

Glow Grazing Is Seasonal

Eating a diet full of glow foods means you are eating in step with nature. Each season, nature gives us the foods we need to prepare us for what lies ahead. In the springtime, we get foods that are cleansing and regenerative, like leafy greens, citrus, and green onion. In the summer, we get foods that are hydrating and cooling—watermelon, cucumber, summer squashes, and berries. In the fall, we indulge in foods that ground us and help prepare our bodies for the cooler months ahead, like beets, soft squashes, and legumes. And in the winter, our biological time for hibernation, we have hard squashes, hearty greens, and grains to keep us warm until the sun comes back!

Health Benefits of Plant-Rich Glow Grazing

A diet rich in whole or minimally processed glow foods provides essential fatty acids, fiber, vitamins, minerals, and phytochemicals that our body needs for radiant energy and optimal function. Many plant-rich glow foods like chia seeds, hemp seeds, and quinoa are complete proteins that provide all the essential amino acids to build muscle tissue. Consuming a diet rich in minimally processed, whole-plant foods also makes managing a healthy weight possible. People who eat mostly plants tend to consume fewer calories and have lower body-mass indexes than those who consume more animal flesh. And glow foods help manage cravings while bringing your body into balance.

Glow foods can protect you from disease, too. Plant-rich diets are linked with decreased risk of heart disease, type 2 diabetes, hypertension, cancer, and other chronic diseases. Personally, I'm a big fan of the cruciferous veggies like broccoli, kale, collards, kohlrabi, mustard greens, and watercress. They contain a substance called indole-3-carbinol (I3C) that inhibits estrogen growth that can cause tumors in breast tissue, protecting the breasts from cysts and cancer.

Fiber also works wonders, limiting estrogen as it binds with the hormone and moves it out of the body. I'm not talking the breakfast cereal on aisle three that claims to contain fiber, but actual vegetable fiber and whole grains. Women who eat a plant-based diet eliminate two to three times more estrogen than their meat-eating counterparts. On top of all this, when you chew these foods, the fiber contained within activates micro sugars, glyconutrients, which have numerous health benefits. Fiber can also reduce the symptoms of PMS.

Plant-based glow grazing also helps combat the effects of oxidants in the body. Oxidants—also known as free radicals—are highly reactive oxygen molecules that cause the breakdown of proteins and enzymes that make up our cells. They occur as a normal part of the body's processes, including metabolism and digestion, but when they are rampant in the system, they can cause problems. Oxidants cause skin dehydration and wrinkle formation as well as a host of degenerative diseases. The main lifestyle causes of oxidant overload include stress, smoking (including secondhand smoke), dietary fat, X-rays, processed foods, industrial toxins, chemical food additives, and too much ultraviolet sun exposure.

Unfortunately, I love spending time in the sun, so that's a hard one for me to avoid. The solution: *anti*oxidants! The major power players include vitamins C, E, and B6; beta-carotene; selenium; magnesium; and glutathione, all of which can be found in glow foods and, in addition to your proper nutrition, you can find these vitamins and minerals in supplement form.

Considering Your Cravings

There is an intelligence rooted in your cells that monitors your physical, emotional, and psychological condition. When it perceives imbalance—malnourishment, dehydration, constipation, stress, duress—it triggers a set of urges designed to restore harmony. These urges are what we know as cravings. We think cravings are universally bad, but often they are the body's way of swinging the pendulum back into balance. When you experience a strong desire for a particular food, it's likely an indication that you are lacking the nutrients that this food offers. For instance, if you are craving bananas, your body may be lacking potassium. Cravings are a primal signal to get us back on track. Appreciate the wisdom of the body, learn to listen to what the body is telling you through your cravings, and pinpoint the underlying need rather than make judgments of yourself for having them.

Here are seven steps to help you tap into the wisdom of your cravings.

- *Step One:* When you feel a desire to eat, observe the emotions that come with it.
- *Step Two:* Drink water. When you feel a craving surface, drink a glass of water and wait 10 minutes to see if the craving subsides. If the craving still lingers or becomes stronger, then you know you're hungry instead of thirsty.

- *Step Three:* Eat a healthy version of the food you crave. A diet of refined foods produces cravings for more of the same. To find your way back to balance, make a gradual transition from your current diet to one dominated by glow foods.

- *Step Four:* Cut the sweets, sugar! When you consume lots of sweets, it makes you crave more sweets as well as the polar opposite, salt. Want to have more sweetness in your life? Try meeting your craving with a little glow time. Take a nice warm bath with candles and lavender essential oil, get your nails done, or go for a massage to meet that emotional need for sweetness in your life.

- *Step Five:* Examine foods and lifestyle factors that may be the deeper source of cravings. If you are stressed at work, at home, or financially, you may find yourself reaching for rich desserts. If you are craving hard candies, popcorn, or crunchy carbs, it may indicate pent-up energy that needs an outlet. Try exercise such as vigorous yoga, a spin class, boot camp, or brisk walks.

- *Step Six:* Question yourself—"If I eat this food, will I feel satisfied?" If the answer is yes, then have a small portion. If the answer is no, try Step One or Two, listed above.

- *Step Seven:* Learn your limits. For many of us, learning to eat when we're hungry is the easy part. We can also learn to tune in to our signals of fullness—and even begin to respect those signals. In order to honor the sensation of fullness, you have to be hungry to begin with so you'll be able to tell when you are not hungry anymore. Food tastes best if you are hungry and have worked up an appetite. Mindful eating allows you to focus on the process of eating.

Let's talk about what your cravings actually mean. The following information is based upon the Traditional Chinese Medicine concept of the five flavors, which defines organ relationships with specific foods and how flavor affects an organ. This is a useful tool to understand where you may have imbalances and what the cravings are saying about your internal state.

- **Sweet** flavors are calming and soothing. Sweets fill an emotional void, and cravings indicate blood-sugar imbalance, the need for emotional equilibrium, or excessive protein consumption.

- **Salty** flavors are softening, and cravings indicate a need for minerals and that you are coping with stress.

- **Bitter** flavors have a drying effect on the body, and cravings indicate a need to cut through fat and the sluggishness of the large intestine.

- **Pungent and spicy** flavors are dispersive, and cravings indicate mucus buildup in the lungs and large intestine. Pungent foods help to induce perspiration and disperse mucus. Spicy cravings may indicate zinc deficiency and that you need help regulating your body temperature.

- **Sour** flavors are astringent and emptying and associated with the liver and gallbladder, and cravings are associated with a chemical imbalance toward acids in the body.

Ancestral Tradition

Each of us comes from a lineage of ancestors who lived in a certain region of the world and were shaped by their environment. Their food choices have become cemented into our heritages and traditions. Today, what we eat (and often what we crave) is linked to those ancestral roots. There is an inherent sense of connection that we all desire on a primal level. For instance, the wildly popular Paleo diet, also known as the "caveman diet," is a movement based on the consumption of foods presumed to be available to our Paleolithic ancestors and includes vegetables, fruits, nuts, roots, and meats. I am not necessarily advocating you follow this diet, but it is one example of people finding their way to honor their ancestral foods. Explore the foods and flavors that you are drawn to and connect with the foods from your heritage, even in the smallest way, like using spice mixtures.

Spicing It Up!

Anyone who knows me knows I love flavor. The key to an abundant and flavorful experience with food is building the taste profile with herbs and spices. When you infuse food with spice, you add a whole other dimension of flavor. But keep in mind, your food is meant to be enhanced by spices and herbs—it shouldn't be dominated by them to the point where you no longer recognize what you're eating. Along with a good salt, adorn your food with flavor, manipulate its texture, and prepare it for joyous consumption. These are the basic seasonings you need in your arsenal in order to turn the ordinary into the impressive in the kitchen.

Black pepper	Curry powder
Cardamom	Garlic
Cinnamon	Ginger
Coriander	Oregano
Crushed red pepper	Smoked paprika
Cumin	Turmeric

Grazing for the Glow

Part of grazing for the glow is fortifying yourself with foods that make you *feel* good. The other part is about eating the foods that make you *look* good! The beauty benefits of a plant-rich diet are unparalleled. Your appearance can be an outer reflection of what is happening inside of your body. Cellular damage from processed foods, stress, and environmental toxins may show up as external symptoms, particularly on the skin, your largest eliminative organ. This accumulation of toxins may result in blemishes, fine lines, and wrinkles.

Eating a diet high in water-laden fruits and vegetables is hydrating for the cells, keeping your skin radiant. Eating for beauty means choosing vital plant foods. Among these are juicy tree fruits that draw their sustenance from the sunlight, but all fruits and vegetables are powerful alkaline agents of change. They dislodge acids and waste from the body, and the water helps carry them out. These foods program our cells. With their high water content, fruits and vegetables hydrate the cells and tissues of the body, removing internal obstructions and revealing the glow from within!

Juicing and Smoothies

Incorporating a variety of whole glow-foods into your diet is important for optimal health. Juice acts like an IV infusion of nutrients, dousing your cells with immediate energy due to its quick assimilation into the bloodstream. Fresh, raw juices relieve the digestive system of the need to expend energy to break down solid food. The less time the body spends digesting and assimilating nutrients, the more time it has to repair and rejuvenate cells and tissues.

Digestion takes a lot of energy and blood flow. When we are thinking about and processing food, it keeps us from being able to be as productive in other areas. Aim for juices with a density of veggies and less fruit so you can help maintain stable blood sugar.

You don't need to renounce the world, move into a cave, and undergo a huge detox to incorporate juice into your daily routine. Juicing is best done on an empty stomach—not a starving one—either in the morning before breakfast or as an afternoon snack and between lunch and dinner. This allows you to fully reap the benefits of the juice because the nutrients are absorbed rapidly.

When making juice, either with a cold press or countertop centrifugal juicer, you are extracting the liquid and most of the nutrients from the more fibrous part of the fruit or vegetable but leaving behind beneficial fiber. Smoothies, on the other hand, are pulverized in a blender with the fiber and its glyconutrients still incorporated. You can have a green smoothie that packs the fiber that juices don't while offering a bit more texture. While smoothies can take a little more time to digest, they can act as a meal replacement. And they are a great option for those who don't want to invest in a juicer or who really want their liquids to take the form of a meal.

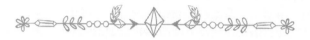

GREEN GLORY

This green juice is nourishing, detoxifying, and refreshing.

> 1 green apple
> ½ cucumber
> ½ fennel bulb
> ½ lemon, peeled
> Handful of kale
> Handful of parsley
> 1 kiwi fruit, peeled
> 1-inch piece of ginger

Wash all the ingredients and process through a juicer. Drink immediately. This recipe can also be prepared as a green smoothie in a high-speed blender.

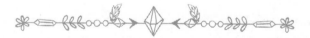

Vitamins and Minerals for Feminine Well-Being

Vitamin A: An antioxidant that helps maintain cell growth and renewal. Found in sweet potatoes, amaranth, carrots, kale, spinach, and Swiss chard.

Vitamin B6: A hormone regulator that also helps to regulate blood sugars, alleviates PMS, and may be useful in relieving symptoms of morning sickness. B6 has also been shown to help with luteal-phase defect. Found in banana, Brussels sprouts, collard greens, garlic, cauliflower, and asparagus.

Vitamin B12: Helps with brain and nervous-system function and formation of DNA and red blood cells. May help to boost the endometrium lining in egg fertilization. Deficiency of B12 may contribute to irregular ovulation. Found in tempeh (fermented soy), nori seaweed, organic vegetables, and animal protein.

B-Complex vitamins: Niacin helps skin retain moisture; biotin strengthens hair and nails. Found in sunflower seeds, wild rice, and sweet potatoes.

Vitamin C: An antioxidant that protects against free radicals and may help with iron absorption. Vitamin C also improves hormone levels and increases fertility in women. Found in lemon, orange, grapefruit, bell peppers, kale, and broccoli.

Calcium: Produces strong bones and helps maintain healthy weight. If women don't ingest enough dietary calcium and vitamin D, the hormones that regulate calcium react negatively with estrogen and progesterone and trigger PMS symptoms. Found in kale, broccoli, watercress, lentils, and almonds.

Vitamin D: Helps the body create sex hormones, which, of course, directly affects ovulation, hormonal balance, and mood. Found in blue-green algae and mushroom varieties like portobello, maitake, morel, button, and shiitake.

Vitamin E: An antioxidant that protects skin from UV damage and protects cells against air pollution. It improves the quality of cervical mucus. Found in sunflower seeds, almonds, spinach, broccoli, and tomato.

Folate: Offsets the toxins in the body by oxygenating our blood with chlorophyll. More oxygen in the blood reduces fatigue and enhances our ability to function throughout the day. Folate helps to prevent neural-tube defects in pregnant women. The dark, chlorophyll-rich leafy greens keep the body youthful, particularly when we tack on some exercise—like kale and collard greens. Folate is also found in pinto beans, garbanzo beans, asparagus, black beans, and kidney beans.

Iron: Oxygenates the blood, promoting your skin's healthy glow. Found in spinach, raisins, quinoa, mushrooms, beans, and nettles.

Vitamin K: Helps the blood clot, which may aid in the reduction of dark under-eye circles. Found in kale, spinach, romaine, Swiss chard, parsley, and broccoli.

Manganese: Helps with proper functioning of the thyroid and governs weight loss, appetite, and metabolism and helps with vitamin absorption. Found in buckwheat, spinach, walnuts, flaxseeds, and cabbage.

Magnesium: Responsible for more than 300 enzyme reactions in the body. Helps cleanse and detoxify the body, eliminates constipation. Relieves achy muscles. Found in broccoli, spinach, Swiss chard, arugula, avocados, bananas, lentils, and chocolate.

Omega-3 fatty acids: Essential fatty acids help fertility by helping to regulate hormones in the body, increasing cervical mucus, promoting ovulation, and increasing blood flow to the reproductive organs. Found in flaxseeds, walnuts, chia seed, borage oil, and algae.

Potassium: Balances pH levels and sodium, which in excess can dry out your skin. Helps combat anxiety and stress, enhances muscle strength, and maintains a healthy blood pressure. Found in Brussels sprouts, pears, dates, chickpeas, coconut water, and bananas.

Silicon: Softens the appearance of wrinkles and makes the skin glow and the eyes shine bright by strengthening connective tissue. Found in cucumber, bell peppers, cabbage, romaine lettuce, tomatoes, and onions.

Zinc: Reduces acne, rebuilds collagen, and may prevent signs of aging and skin damage such as wrinkles and stretch marks. Helps to maintain reproductive balance. Found in raw chocolate, pumpkin seeds, green peas, and sesame seeds.

Learn to Cook for You!

They say a way to a man's heart is through his stomach. And, sure, it's nice when you can show off your culinary expertise to impress others. But do it for yourself first—not because it makes you a more attractive mate or looks good on your resume! And certainly not simply because it will make your mother happy. Cook for you because it will increase your sense of self-satisfaction and self-reliance.

We've become a culture obsessed by convenience. The time it takes to do something as simple as cutting up fruit is seen as an inconvenience. It's become widely acceptable to order out all the time.

I don't know when it became cool to rely solely upon others for your nourishment. There are only two instances where that is acceptable: when you are sick and when you're an infant. Once you get to an age where you can start banging some pots and pans in the kitchen, it's time for you to learn how to cook! I started to teach my son the value of nutrition through cooking exercises when he was two years old. Using age-appropriate methods and tasks, he learned to cut up his bananas, how to peel an orange, how to make ratatouille, and more. But if you didn't learn when you were younger, now is a great time to enroll in a cooking academy and take some classes. I highly recommend a knife-skills class followed by basic meal prep to start.

With new "health food" restaurants springing up everywhere, it's easy to eat out and assume you're getting healthier options on your plate and in your belly. But you need to be able to nourish yourself first and know what's going into your body. You can't monitor that through takeout or eating out, no matter how clean you think it is. I'm not saying you can't order in your favorite sushi or Indian fare every now and again, but to know the menu by heart and have the number in your speed dial is a little excessive. When you prepare a meal from scratch, you will feel connected to it and want to savor it and share it.

Your Glow Bowl

I love one-bowl meals because they are simple to make, nourishing, and delicious. Although I enjoy sharing recipes, this is more of a glow-bowl-guide, providing you with some suggestions for how to build a great bowl and experiment with what works best for you.

PROTEIN
Lentils, beans, nuts, seeds, quinoa, chili, hummus, tempeh

VEGETABLES (Raw/Cooked):
Beets, arugula, spinach, pumpkin, squashes, radishes, sprouts, dandelion, watercress, raddichio, mizuna, mache, tomatoes

PSEUDO GRAINS
Amaranth, wild rice, buckwheat, quinoa

FATS
Avocado, nuts, seeds, cold-pressed oils

PROBIOTIC (Fermented) FOODS:
Kimchi, sauerkraut, pickled vegetables

glow tips for
Successful Healthful Cooking

Practice the power of your intention. Our intentions are so important. Prepare food from a positive space. Food is sacred; you should feel honored to be able to prepare food and eat it. Feeling thankful for what you have and sharing what you have with others will not only make you feel good, it will make your food good. Play music. Think positive thoughts. Get your family involved in the process. You may want to set up a kitchen altar. It can be a small shelf with enough space for a small vase or incense holder, perhaps a picture of an ancestor. When you prepare to cook, light a candle or some incense and be present.

Cook with others. If cooking is new for you and you experience some trepidation in kitchen, then invite a few friends over to help you execute your menu. It will make the process fun, and time will fly by. You can serve each other and share in the burden of cleaning up the mess afterward as well. You can also host a pantry party where everyone brings ingredients to make a dish, snack, or condiment, along with containers to store the excess.

Engage in sensual food preparation. Use all your senses in food preparation. The culinary arts are the only art form whereby you experience the materials on all sensory levels—while creating it and then in the finished work! Be mindful of how you are engaging your senses. Smell the ingredients while you cook, taste the dish every step of the way, and listen to the sizzle of the infused oil.

Cook today, eat tomorrow. Batch cooking, or planning your meals for the week and cooking a surplus ahead, makes certain that you always have something healthy on hand. On a day when your schedule is light, plan out the meals for the following week and make your grocery list. Go shopping that day, and when you get home, start prepping your meals for the week ahead, whether that's peeling veggies and cutting them up so they are ready for a stir-fry, making a batch of quinoa to last the week, or preparing your own salad dressings and making snacks.

Practice intuitive cooking. Allow creativity to flow in the kitchen. It's not all about recipes; it's about sensing what is right for you, your palate, and your mood. Try preparing something without a recipe and see what happens. If you engage your senses while eating, you will develop wisdom that tells you what is in the food. You won't need to follow so many steps, giving you more space to celebrate food.

Top Foods to Avoid

Certain foods just aren't good for us. Your glow power comes from taking care of yourself and feeding your body what it needs to thrive so you can maintain a vibrant lifestyle. Examine your current diet to see how much of the following it includes and start to adjust your intake accordingly.

Coffee. I know you don't want to hear this, but America's most widely used drug is coffee. It's highly disruptive to the nervous system and extremely acidifying. Coffee wreaks havoc on your blood-sugar levels and increases stress on the body.
Try instead: green tea, matcha, or herbal-tea blends.

Dairy. Hold up, wait—don't eat that mac and cheese! You should be weaned by now, girlfriend. Dairy interferes with our hormonal signals and a multitude of disorders have been attributed to it—reproductive and otherwise. Plus, it causes weight gain. How do you think a 70-pound calf gets to weigh 500 pounds at a year old? By drinking its mother's milk.
Try instead: almond milk, vegan cheeses, or vegan patés

Alcohol. You may like your margarita or gin and tonic during a night out on the town, but over time, alcohol acts as a depressant and depletes the feel-good hormone serotonin. Most of my clients who eliminate it see a dramatic shift in their weight. This isn't a death sentence—you can still go out at night. But choose how often you drink. You'll get used to how good it feels to rise up in the morning with clarity, without the haze of the liquid fire from the night before.

Try instead: wine spritzers, sparkling mineral water with a little lime and mint, or a virgin drink option

Artificial sweeteners. Poison alert! Steer clear of artificial sweeteners, including those in gum and mints. Healthier alternatives include low-glycemic sweeteners. If you need to chew gum, try xylitol gum.

Try instead: maple syrup, stevia, or honey

White sugar. Sugar depresses the immune system for up to six hours after consumption. It creates a dependency on sweets and erodes the body from within.

Try instead: dates, fruits, maple syrup, honey, or sweet potato

Processed foods. It's best to start eliminating processed foods like chips, breads, and pastries now. Whatever your go-to food is, ask yourself if there is a healthier version.

Try instead: flax crackers, nut bars, fruit, or smoothies

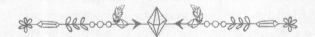

RITUAL:
SIPPING GOLDEN MILK TEA

My friend, designer and actor Waris Ahluwalia, uses tea as an entry point for mindfulness. When tea is served hot, in an open ceramic cup, we have no choice but to move slowly and patiently. Tea stops us in our tracks and brings us into the present moment. It's also a wonderful alternative if you are looking to reduce your coffee intake. This lightly spiced golden elixir (which is similar in flavor to chai) is packed with anti-inflammatory properties and loaded with anti-oxidants thanks to a dose of peppery turmeric. It's a soothing blend that will quickly become one of your favorites.

> 1 cup unsweetened non-dairy milk, preferably coconut milk or almond milk
> 1 (3-inch) cinnamon stick
> 1 (1-inch) piece turmeric, unpeeled, thinly sliced, or ½ teaspoon dried turmeric
> 1 (½-inch) piece ginger, unpeeled, thinly sliced
> 1 tablespoon maple syrup
> 1 tablespoon virgin cold-pressed coconut oil
> ¼ teaspoon whole black peppercorns
> Ground cinnamon (for serving)

Whisk the non-dairy milk, cinnamon stick, turmeric, ginger, maple syrup, coconut oil, peppercorns, and 1 cup water in a small saucepan; bring to a low boil. Reduce heat and simmer until flavors have blended, about 10 minutes. Strain through a fine-mesh sieve into mugs and top with a dash of cinnamon.

Golden milk can be made 5 days ahead and stored in an airtight container in the fridge. Warm before serving.

Sit still with your cup and sip your golden milk. Focus on being present to the experience you are having, savoring the layers of flavor.

The Glow Grazer's Dinner Party

Food is the foundation of our world cultures; it is tied to tradition, ceremony, rituals, and most important, community. And yet we have lost so much of the daily celebratory magic around food in this country. In certain parts of Europe, like France and Spain, meals are still considered times when connection is key and everything else stops. I invite you to create that experience of communing with others around food.

For this exercise, you will prepare a meal for friends or loved ones—not a traditional meal around a holiday, per se, just a meal where you prepare the elements and invite others to join you for the simple reason that you love them. From the shopping list to meal prep, from candlelight and décor to serving the food, I want you to pay attention to the details and make this a special evening. You might send beautiful invites or evites. Perhaps you could have a theme. A successful dinner party is one of the greatest achievements that the home chef can claim. Entertaining can be stressful, but don't let that stop you from hosting a night to remember. These glow guidelines will help guarantee your success and make the night more manageable!

Steer clear of the maiden voyage. It might seem like a good idea to try a new and exciting recipe for your friends, but you don't want to discover 45 minutes before guests arrive that you were supposed to slow roast the tomatoes for six hours before pureeing them into the sauce. Stick to something that you have tried out before.

Make as much as far in advance as you can. Think of how precious those moments are before the doorbell rings. You should be able to pour yourself a glass of wine, put on a dress, and light some candles instead of running around the kitchen like you're a contestant on *Iron Chef*.

Triple-check the ingredient list. Even if you've made this eggplant Napoleon 20 times or more, it's still a good idea to remind yourself of its specifics, like the fresh parsley and sage you forgot to buy last time.

Get on board with **mise en place.** Have all the ingredients out and ready to go before you start cooking. It may seem very Martha Stewart, but it takes less of your time to get things done if you aren't frazzled. This is also a great way to discover whether you are short on ginger or lemons in time to buy more.

Start cooking earlier than you think you should. We always think we have more time than we do. Guests are generally happy to wait on dinner, but not until 11 P.M. (Unless, of course, you live in Madrid. Then that timing is on point!)

Take guests' dietary restrictions into consideration. I have fallen victim to dinners where I am relegated to eating salad, bread, and wine because the hosts didn't consider veggie options. You're not a restaurant, so you don't have to go crazy, but make sure you have enough options for everyone.

Make no apologies. Did you overcook when roasting the sweet potatoes? So what? Own it. No one has ever left a dinner party thinking, "I wish she'd apologized for the okra being soggy."

Make a playlist. My son is a deejay, so I am always hooked up with the right music. Background music makes all the difference. Remember to keep it just loud enough so guests can enjoy it but still engage in conversation.

Use cloth napkins. It's a dinner party, damn it! You can do the whole paper-towel, take-out-container balancing act the next day when your guests are gone. Don't have any cloth napkins? You can find affordable ones online or in any common store like Target.

Take care of the basics. If it's an essential item, like ice for the cocktails, you don't want to be left in the lurch if a guest who has offered to bring something doesn't show up. Make sure you have all the things you need on hand.

Invite the right mix of people. It might be tempting to introduce all your favorite friends to each other at once, but if you are the only thing they have in common, the evening might feel more like a mixer than a proper dinner party. Take a note from recipes: add new elements a little bit at a time.

Be seated with your guests. Plan the menu and the service so that you're able to enjoy the meal, too. You deserve a chance to eat! Besides, no one wants to be at a dinner party where the host spends most of the evening urging people to eat while he or she stirs something on the stove.

Create atmosphere! Light some candles. Atmosphere is what makes a dinner party a party. Your tablescape doesn't have to be over-the-top, but it should look nice. Candles are inexpensive, readily available, and a great place to start.

Provide dessert. Whether it's a beautiful fruit platter or something homemade, dessert is a good way to begin to wind down the party and transition to whatever is next. Perhaps you can serve dessert in a different location to shift the energy.

Don't leave dirty dishes overnight. This was engrained in me as a kid. My mom always left the kitchen clean. Make sure to start the cleanup before bed. That Dutch oven will be impossible to clean the next day. And you'll be so happy to wake up to a clean kitchen.

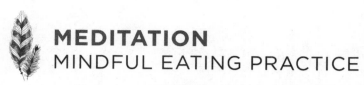

MEDITATION
MINDFUL EATING PRACTICE

You can use your mealtimes as a way to nourish yourself physically and spiritually. When you place a piece of fruit into your mouth, be aware and focus on the food. If you're focused on your work, you're not eating mindfully, you're multitasking. Here is a meditation to help ground you in the moment and focus you on eating.

Take a seat at the dining table. Sit up tall with your feet grounded beneath you and gaze at the food before you. If you are joined by friends, family, or people around the table, or if you are eating alone, notice how nice it feels to slow down, sit, and be present before a meal. Breathe deeply, inhale the aroma of your food, and exhale. Close your eyes. Give thanks for your meal. As you sit, think about how many hands and hearts have been involved in bringing your food to your plate. Feel your heart warm with gratitude for all the work that went into manifesting your meal. Your food contains not only nutrients but cosmic energy. It was made with sunshine, wind, rain, and earth. It may have been harvested by people you will never meet or have a chance to thank. Bless the hands of those who worked the land that produced your food. Pay attention to each spoonful or bite, knowing that it is a gift from the Universe. When you chew, stay with the awareness that the entire Universe is present within each bite. Take your time and eat slowly and intentionally, nourishing yourself with each breath and each bite.

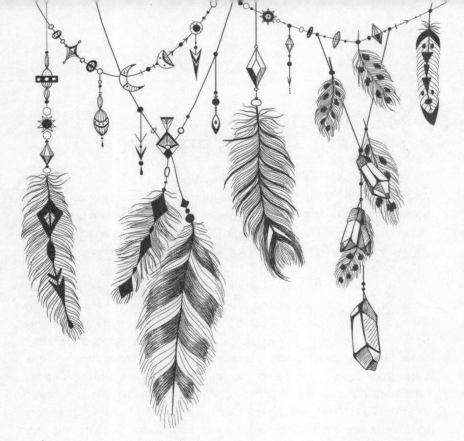

"*If a woman sits with folded hands in her lap for a few minutes every day, and feels she is a container so vast that she contains the whole Universe, she will never feel weak or have any problems. There is nothing beyond woman except God.*"

– Yogi Bhajan

glow motion

*"I think that training is the key, definitely,
and I devoted my life to it."*

~ MISTY COPELAND, THE FIRST AFRICAN-AMERICAN
PRINCIPAL DANCER WITH THE AMERICAN BALLET THEATER

Incorporating movement into our daily lives enhances our glow, "intunes" us with our GPS, and sets us on a path to achieving our purpose and our best selves.

Movement is a big part of dialing up your glow power and will help you stay on course with your mission. Moving your body builds heat that creates strength and flexibility, as well as an opening for a mental or spiritual breakthrough. I can't tell you how many people have come up to me and shared how they came up with their million-dollar idea after yoga class or how a solution to a huge problem was born after a three-mile run.

Movement helps to open our creative portal. For me, that means yoga. Yoga can be made accessible to almost everyone but may not *resonate* with everyone. I encourage you to try it if you can, but if it's not for you, then find *your* yoga. Find what brings you peace—in nature, on a bike, or in the gym. It may be kickboxing, fencing, tae kwon do, or salsa dancing.

If you have sustained any injuries that have resulted in your physical movement being severely restricted, perhaps try integrating a mild stretching practice or incorporating a rehabilitative practice a few days a week to strengthen the supporting muscles and connective tissue around the injuries. If you find the thought of exercise overwhelming, no matter the reason, remember it's all about baby steps.

If going to a gym is frightening, how about subscribing to a fitness app, online program, or videos on YouTube that you can start at home where you feel safe. It helps to have motivators. Perhaps a friend can join you in your workouts, which you can keep under 45 minutes so you stay committed. When you feel more comfortable, attend a group fitness class and bring a buddy along for moral support. Note that you should consult with your physician first before adding any drastically different exercise into your routine.

Glow motion is about engaging in movement that feels amazing. It's about honoring your sacred body. It is about receiving the gift.

Intention

The intent behind your chosen movement activity has to stem from a place of nourishment and nurturing. If you look beneath the usual goals of losing weight—having a nice backside, tight abs, or sexy arms—you'll see that the real intention beneath the surface is to feel good, content, uplifted, and energized. Simply reframing the language around our exercise and choosing to focus on its positive health and wellness benefits rather than an outcome in pounds or inches allows us to be gentle on ourselves and less competitive. It invites a positive starting place.

I love the intenSati method that incorporates yoga, dance, and affirmations, developed by fitness and lifestyle visionary Patricia Moreno. It combines functional movements with affirmations like "I am powerful now" and a movement that illustrates power. During her class, the focus is on learning the repetitive choreography, which is aligned with upbeat music, and proclaiming the affirmations out loud. It's about intention and movement. I feel blissful after Patricia's classes, like I just received a pep talk that will motivate me for the entire day. Similarly, when I take a ride with fitness evangelist and senior Soul-Cycle instructor Angela Davis, I am coasting afterward. Angela, who was an elite Olympic track athlete, infuses the drive, intensity, and focus it took to be the best on the track into her spiritual and soulful class. She uses the power of intention, affirmation, and music as she coaches clients through a ride that transforms their lives. While it's nice to have superstar teachers lead you though group fitness classes, you can transform your workouts on your own.

You can bring this practice of affirming yourself in your activities no matter what you do. Get clear about what activities feel most aligned with your energy and use positive language as you engage in them. During a squat sequence, you might repeat the affirmation "I am powerful." For a push-up sequence, you might try, "I am strong, I am bold, my own strength I can hold."

Do What You Like

To allow the intention of your movement practice to unfold, you have to be in love with what you are doing. If you don't love lifting weights but force yourself to do it because you should, then your head won't be in the game. When you're not present and engaged, your mind is free to focus on other things that have no business crowding your thoughts, such as your dry cleaning, your taxes, or how big your thighs look. And if you dislike the activity, you are also setting your body up for a stressful experience rather than a stress release.

Be Engaged

Exercise is not just about fitting some into your busy day. It's about being engaged in the process and experience. Movement is a part of your self-care practice and, as such, you need to make space for it. How can you reframe your movement practice from something you need to cross off your to-do list to a sustainable self-care practice? To figure out your ideal practice, sit still in a quiet space, close your eyes, and breathe. Ask yourself: "How will I choose to move my body today? What moves and uplifts me? What makes me feel good?"

There is no one perfect movement; everyone is different and has different needs. Tune in to what makes you feel radiant. Rather than watching CNN on the treadmill at the gym, connect with your body in a meaningful way that also yields feel-good results.

The Sister System

Much like the buddy system, in the sister system, you employ one or two friends who share the same passion, or challenges, around movement. A sister needs to be someone who is motivating, who will hold you accountable, and whom you will hold accountable in turn. You will share your fitness progress with each other, set goals together, do movement together, and celebrate when you succeed! Find the right time to work out together so you can maximize your results and stay committed. Some examples of movement perfectly suited to the sister system include jogging, dance class, SoulCycle, or a boot-camp type program.

Be Prepared

Success on your fitness and wellness journey largely depends on you being prepared. Make sure you have the gear you need to succeed—whether that's new yoga pants, proper running shoes, a swim cap, or a water bottle—so you feel ready for the activity you're embarking upon.

Enter the Mind-set

There will always be an excuse or obstacles that keep you from exercising. To stay in the mind-set, we need commitment.

Visualize your fulfilled goal. Really take yourself to a place where you see yourself attaining the goal. Focus on the feeling and map the experience so you have a mental blueprint.

Treat yourself. When you slip from the routine, don't punish yourself; just commit to starting again and getting back on course. But when you have committed to your training plan or exercise schedule and have achieved a milestone, celebrate yourself. You might get a new pair of running shoes, purchase a new luxury candle, or indulge yourself with some glow time and book a full body massage.

Set a date. Commit to your workout or movement practice by scheduling it into your day. Whether you use a manual planner or plug your weekly schedule into your phone or computer, these appointments with yourself are just as important as any other meeting or task you have planned.

Make a motivation mix. Playing upbeat music while you engage in fitness activity will motivate you to keep going. Create playlists that correspond with warm-up, high-energy, restorative, and cool-down elements of your practice.

Splurge on yourself. Invest in some quality workout gear. If you dress in something you love, you will feel more confident on the mat, in the gym, on the bike, or wherever your workout takes you.

Movement Reboot

If you need to make your way back to balance or if you need to ground yourself, these three fundamental tuning exercises are great for hitting control-alt-delete and rebooting yourself. You can do these movements anywhere.

Just breathe. Spend a few minutes each day, either in silence or with a dope playlist, paying attention to your breath. You can simply observe your natural breathing or choose a breathing pattern. Here are some examples:

1. Receive a breath through the nose, inhaling for 4 counts. Pause and hold for 1 to 2 counts. Release through the mouth for 4 counts.

2. Receive a breath through the nose, inhaling for 5 counts. Pause and hold for 5 counts. Release through the nose for 5 counts.

3. Receive a breath through the nose, inhaling for 4 counts and envisioning the word *sat.* Pause and hold for as long as feels comfortable. Release through the nose and envision the word *naam.* (*Sat naam* means I AM, or "my true self.")

Stretch it out. Stretching helps us find space in our body, promoting a balance of strength and flexibility that chemically translates into clarity and perspective in the mind and consciousness. Think of a stretch like that of a yawning cat finding extension in its full body. When you stretch, your muscles, connective tissue, joints, and organs get an internal massage. It's a way to connect and understand what is happening in the body and perhaps what it needs as well. Through stretching, you become aware of tightness in certain areas as well as tension and holding patterns that have lodged themselves in your body. Explore your movement vocabulary on the mat with these stretches:

1. **Toe-ga.** This is yoga for your toes. This is especially good for those of us who love to wear heels! Really massage your feet. Roll the soles of your feet on a tennis ball. Flex and extend, and then point and straighten your feet. Much of our structural misalignment occurs because of our feet being overworked.

2. **Cat-cow posture.** Get on all fours in a tabletop position, and on the inhale, roll the hips forward and send the tailbone back behind you for cow position. Then on the exhale, round your shoulders and spine, moving through cat position. This is one of the most basic yoga postures, and it is key to a flexible and healthy spine. It's also a great way to warm up the major joints in the body.

3. **Heart opener.** Standing on your knees or in hero's pose, sitting on your heels with shins pressed into the floor and stretching out your quads, take your arms behind your back and interlace your fingers, drawing your shoulder blades together. Receive a breath and open your chest. Hold this position for five breaths and then bow forward over your legs. With your fingers still interlaced, reach your arms overhead.

Quickies! Lack of sleep, overwork, and stress can take a toll on your lymphatic system and nervous system. This can cause sluggishness and interferes with the natural functions of your body. Moving around in quick bursts can counteract that sluggishness. It's like a spring cleaning for your body. Old sediment gets lifted and eventually cleared out through sweat, urine, or stool, paving the way for fresh, clear pathways, new opportunities, and nourishing life patterns. Here are some ways to move your body quickly:

Hybrid workouts. We have all heard of the benefits of mixing up our exercise routines through cross-training, from preventing burnout and injuries to maximizing results. Find simple solutions like cardio tennis and speed walking with intervals.

Plank and crawl. Plank pose, or push-up position, is a challenge for everyone. Try "crawling" in a horizontal position from plank (push-up position) or forearm plank pose by driving your right knee to the right elbow, then extending the leg back to plank and switching to the opposite side. Repeat the plank crawls in this position for a minimum of 20 counts.

Blast-off. Is there a staircase that you can incorporate into your workout reboot? Near my house, there is a subway station with a very long staircase that I always opt to sprint—unless I am wearing heels, of course. Quick bursts of movement get your blood circulating and activate a testosterone release that keeps thyroid levels in balance, triggering the burning of fat.

Jumping to it. Jump rope is an amazing full-body workout. It's a favorite in boxing gyms for warm-ups, and there are even hour-long jump-rope classes! You can turn on your favorite dance music or hip hop, get pumped up, and jump. There are weighted ropes that can challenge you more if you want to really work the arms and back muscles. Don't worry if you're not so great at it at first. You'll get the hang of it. My favorite is jumping rope in Central Park on the bridle path in the early morning.

Your Glow-Flow Yoga Practice

Yoga has both a sole purpose and a soul purpose, and it is to unite the mind and body, reintegrating universal consciousness with your individual consciousness. When you practice the elements of asana (yoga posture) and *pranayama* (breath work) on a frequent basis, reintegration occurs. There are many health benefits associated with a regular yoga practice, including reduced stress, increased flexibility of the joints, improved muscle tone, balanced hormones, lower blood pressure, a draining of the lymphatic system, weight loss, and improved respiration, energy, and vitality.

Don't worry if you have never practiced yoga before—yoga is for everyone of every age, shape, and size. Most studios have a beginner's track that you can sign up to take before joining the general classes so you can get familiar with the movements and proper body positions. I love online yoga classes as an option for those who are far too busy to show up to a yoga class but still want to experience the benefits at home or in their offices.

How we begin our day can have a huge impact on how it unfolds. When we start our day with intention, conscious movement, rhythmic breathing, and a focused mind, we're setting ourselves up for excellence. You may not always have 90 minutes for a yoga class, but combining some postures in a quick sequence can help you make the best of whatever time you have on hand. Remember to set up your space with whatever you need to get grounded for these next few minutes—music, a candle, incense, or even simply opening the window for fresh air.

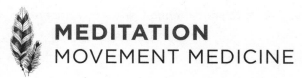

MEDITATION
MOVEMENT MEDICINE

Movement meditation is mindful and intentional, free and fluid movement that heals. It's an opportunity to connect to what's happening within your body and move in a way that feels natural and unrestricted.

Prepare for the meditation by setting the mood for the space with low lighting from drawn curtains or candlelight. Set the right music so you have an inspired flow; I suggest something instrumental and repetitive in nature so you aren't mentally connected to the lyrics. Light incense and set your intention, or a seed goal—one focused around what you need before you begin. There may be a single word that comes to the surface when you set your intention, like *love*. You might use that word to inform the music and help lead into your movement. This meditation is about freedom of movement, so do whatever feels good to you. This meditation is most effective when practiced for a minimum of 10 minutes.

Start in a seated position with your eyes closed and focus on the breath. While moving in sync with the music, begin hip swivels in a circular motion. From there, you may want to move gracefully onto your hands and knees, rolling your hips, moving in a feline manner, articulating your spine. While your knees are still on the mat, lift your upper body and create waves with your torso and arms. Be free with your movement. Make your way to standing while moving through low squats. Give yourself what you need to work out any tightness or tension in the body. Move in spiral forms, creating rhythm, ritual, and repetition. Move around the space however your body wants. Start asking yourself, "What do I need?" And allow your body to answer through fluid movement. When you are ready to bring the movement meditation to a close, start to slow down and make smaller movements and find your way back to the floor into a child's pose or a seated position with palms positioned facing up over your knees. With your eyes closed, tune in to your body and notice how you are feeling. Observe your heart rate, your breath, observe your disposition. Return to your intention, and when you are ready, open your eyes.

Glow-Flow Yoga Sequence

This 15-minute vinyasa flow is easy to fit into your morning routine. The following postures warm up the physical body, encourage detoxification and blood flow, and help you build a connection with your breath, easing you into a positive mind-set for an abundant day.

Grounding: Start in a seated position, cross-legged with hands in *anjali* mudra or prayer position, palms pressed lightly together at the heart center. Close your eyes and set an intention for the day.

Your intention should be a short reflection, a positive affirming dedication, or simply a word that serves to inspire you toward a more uplifted state of being.

Cat/cow: Come to hands and knees with your shoulders, elbows, and wrists in alignment, fingers spread wide, and your hips over your knees. Inhale, gaze forward, and tilt the pelvis back, lifting the tailbone and keeping the heart lifted as the belly dips (cow pose).

Exhale to cat pose, pressing the mat away as you draw your navel up toward your spine and tuck the chin toward your chest, rounding and stretching your back. Keep flowing between the two poses.

Plank: From hands and knees, step one foot back and then the other so you're in a push-up position. You want the body to be in a long line, feeling the crown of the head lengthen forward as the tail and heels lengthen back. Keep your shoulders over your wrists, and draw your navel up toward the spine. Engage the thighs and hold the pose for 30 seconds while breathing.

Downward-facing dog: Place hands shoulder-width apart on the mat, fingers spread wide. Glide the hips up and back, and start off with the knees bent so you can work on lengthening your tail/spine. Straighten one leg at a time, checking out how the hamstrings feel as you settle both heels toward the ground. If your body is a little stiff in the morning, you can keep your knees bent. Hold the pose for at least five deep breaths.

Low lunge: Keep the core switched on as you step the right foot forward (from downward-facing dog) between the feet. Lower the back knee onto the mat with the front knee extending just over the ankle. Sweep the arms up overhead, fingers reaching toward the sky. Lengthen the tailbone down toward the mat and draw the lower ribs and lower belly in to support the lower back.

Feel levity and stay for at least five deep breaths.

High lunge: Repeat the steps for the previous pose, but this time, keep the back knee off the mat. Really engage through the back leg and feel it power you through the pose. Keep your fingers active and energized as you reach up overhead.

Goddess squats: Pivot your feet so you are facing sideways on your mat and have a slight turnout with your feet. Straighten your legs and inhale, and bring your arms up overhead. Exhale, bend your knees, and open your arms into a *U* position for squats. Your knees should be directly over your ankles and thighs as parallel as possible to the floor. Move through a sequence of squats for 20 counts.

Warrior I transition: Pivot the feet so the right foot turns forward and the left heel drops down to the mat. Bend your front knee with arms raised forward and alongside your head in Warrior I position. Hold for five deep breaths, then step back to plank position.

After holding plank position for five breaths, repeat the sequence—downward-facing dog, low lunge, high lunge, squats, and warrior I—on the opposite side.

After completing the postures on both sides, step back to downward-facing dog.

Child's pose: From downward-facing dog, bend your knees to the floor. Center your breath and turn your awareness inward. Spread your knees apart while keeping your big toes touching. Rest your buttocks on your heels. If your hips are tight, keep your knees and thighs together. Your heart and chest should rest between or on top of your thighs. Allow your forehead to come to the floor. Keep your arms long and extended, palms facing down. For deeper relaxation, bring your arms back to rest alongside your thighs with your palms facing up, ready to receive.

At the end of this sequence, it's nice to stand or sit quietly with the hands in *anjali* mudra, or prayer position, returning your focus to the intention or word that you cultivated at the beginning of the practice. Reconnect with that positive anchoring intention. After a few moments, gently open your eyes, smile, and let your intention carry you through the day.

THE TRUTH IS A FORM OF MAGIC.

the threshold

HOLY GLOW!

"The only permission, the only validation, and the only opinion that matters in our quest for greatness is our own."

~ STEVE MARABOLI, *UNAPOLOGETICALLY YOU:*
REFLECTIONS ON LIFE AND THE HUMAN EXPERIENCE

Welcome to the final stretch. You're about to cross the threshold and emerge with something you didn't have when you started. You have harnessed your living rituals and can use them to amplify your power source—your GPS. You are fully ready to take this journey on your own. You've learned to listen to the whispers. You know what you're calling into your orbit. You know enough about yourself at this point to bring anything you want into fruition.

To develop unbridled self-love that is not based upon external validation is a challenging task. In these pages, we've taken that challenge full on. From an early age, we have been conditioned to base our self-worth on how much attention we get, money we make, and hierarchal positions we hold. We've been taught that other women and their successes are a threat to our own shine. We judge ourselves constantly based on outside forces. You are a reservoir of light. Forget what anyone else has told you about yourself that has dismantled part of your self-worth. In spite of all the noise, the likes, the pain, the praise, the challenges and triumphs, the hurdles and standing ovations, you are already crowned. You are crystalline in your queenliness.

Step into your glow power. Revel in the gentle sway of a hammock, stop to talk to strangers, say yes to risk, and turn your walk into a run. You are on a velvet-curtained center stage. Light up a new path with your stilettos and climb higher and go farther. You are dazzling through and through. You are full of seed potential.

Wombifesting is all about tuning inward, surrendering, and creating a vacuum to draw to yourself all that you desire. You have *evoked* and called in your mission, clearing any blocks to your greatness. You have *ignited* your path and trusted the wisdom of the sacred feminine cycles and divine timing. You have *embodied* the principles of this lifestyle to maximize your glow.

You're ready to take the leap, my friend! I only have a few more pieces of wisdom for you as you fully step out onto the path of owning your glow.

Faith It till You Make It

When you are aspiring to achieve a goal, when you are positioning yourself for something you aren't yet ready for but are calling it in, you aren't faking. You're becoming. There is a difference, and the hustle is real.

You are rising in consciousness, in spirit, in flesh, and aligning your actions so they are pursuant with that goal or experience you are striving toward. It's knowing that what you long for on a soul level is making its way into your orbit. You're moving with faith.

"Faith it till you make it" is a divine process of creation vibration. It's a conscious choice to become ready for what awaits you. Your steady readiness to lean into the unknown and walk in faith signals the Universe that you are ready for more blessings. Remember, all things grow in the dark. Own your glow, and it will light your path along the way.

From Dreaming to Doing

Focused action, consistent belief, and trust in your process will help you achieve anything. Dream, but then start with an annual scope, and set intentions and plans into motion. Quarterly, check in and see how you are tracking against your goals. Do you need to make any adjustments? Are you still feeling aligned with the vision? Monthly, make a plan and map out what lies ahead and how you are addressing the goals in bite-sized pieces. Weekly, take action aligned with your intentions. What are your priorities this week? How will you maintain well-being? Daily, focus and remind yourself of your creative force.

Soul scribe on the following:

Dreams I am holding for self-love _____

_____

_____

Dreams I have for my myself and community _____

_____

_____

Dreams I have for my abundant career _____

_____

_____

_____

Dreams I have for love and relationships _____

_____

_____

Dreams I have for health and well-being _____

_____

_____

How will I live my life accordingly and align action with new choices that support these dreams? _____

_____

_____

_____

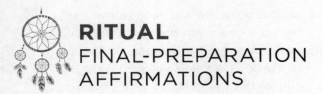

RITUAL
FINAL-PREPARATION AFFIRMATIONS

This ritual is meant as a final preparation as you start out on your own path. Soul-scribe your affirmations so they are fresh in your mind and ready for you to act upon.

Evoke the ability to make healthy choices and create more beauty in your life. Write at least one mantra or affirmation that will help keep you focused around your goals for self-care and self-love.

Ignite the ability to harness your creativity and adjust your mind-set. Write at least one mantra to help keep you focused and inspired while sweeping away self-doubt and honoring your work, creativity, and feminine edge.

Embody the power of your conscious words and intentions, not by force but by grace. It's a conscious choice to become ready for what awaits you. Write at least one mantra that will help you be the light, that will help you hold your vision high and never lose sight no matter how dark it gets along the way.

My New Motto

A motto is a short expression of an important guiding principle. What's the motto for your movement? Each of us has sacred magic that we were born with that is a gift for the world, and it's our job to sprinkle that magic onto the world. What's your big leap? If there is no risk, there is no real reward.

*My new motto is:*_____

_____

_____

_____

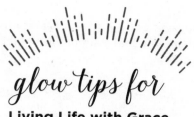

glow tips for
Living Life with Grace

Live inside the silver lining. You are anointed. You have been chosen to walk a unique path that you are meant to unfold. You are precious. See everything as shiny, embrace gratitude, and find the silver lining in every situation. Know that the silver lining stays polished with positive thinking and your engagement with gratitude will help you to see the brilliance and blessing in everything.

Be cozy in your own skin. You want to feel good in your body and spirit. Love your shape, your peaks, and your valleys.

Embrace the energy of ease. Seek relationships and circumstances that support ease and agility, that give you room to breathe and grow. The energy of ease is all about allowance. Rather than forcing something, *let* it move naturally so you can experience more abundance, connection, and flow.

Lose control. Relinquish the need to have dominion over everything. Losing control is about surrender, tuning in to the rhythms, and allowing yourself to be at ease.

Own your pleasure. If you aren't having fun, it doesn't count. We need to become unapologetic about our pleasure. Go out and do what inspires you, as it will energize you along the journey.

Be present. This moment, this time and place, is blessed. This configuration will never occur again in the same way. Honor what's going on for you right now.

Jet-set. Travel allows us to gain perspective on life and explore the internal landscape within. Take that much-needed vacation alone or with girlfriends!

Dare to dream. Go to a special place where you do your best work, where you feel inspired and in the flow. Use your creative freedom and get to work on your dreams.

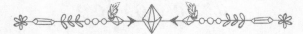

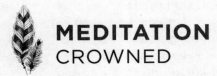

MEDITATION
CROWNED

This final meditation is focused upon visualizing your highest self, the best iteration of you. Find a quiet place of peace and calm, whether that's in your bedroom, in your office, or on a park bench. Set aside a minimum of 5 minutes or, if you regularly engage in a mindfulness practice, 15 minutes may be a perfect window for this exercise. The goal is to increase a sense of overall well-being—so sit for as along or as short as feels comfortable to you.

Become present, feeling the support of life around and within you. As you begin to bring your attention to your breath, notice your body relax. Allow peace to fill every part of you as you move even more deeply into the quiet with focus on a sacred word such as love, peace, grace, *or* I Am.

I invite you to gently close your eyes and focus within on your breath, your life force. On the inhale, feel the belly expand, and on the exhale, feel everything move toward the middle of your body.

Receive a breath and expand for five counts, allowing the breath to swirl as you retain it for five counts.

Exhale and release the breath for five long counts.

Inhale and receive courage and faith.

Exhale and release doubt and worry.

Repeat to yourself silently or out loud:
The light of love surrounds me

The energy of love enfolds me

The power of love protects me
The presence of love is within me

Sit in the peace of meditation and open to timeless holiness. You are a sacred vessel to the future. Staying quiet, relaxed, and simply being in deeper attunement, know that you are holy, you are filled with light. Feel the elements of the ambient landscape all around you. You are a part of this cosmic matrix. All is well. Listen to the wisdom of the whispers. Release all seeds of self-doubt and plant seeds for your fruitful future. Place your hands upon your heart center and take a deep bow, saluting yourself and your seed potential. When you focus on what you believe, programmed limiting beliefs surface as well. What could be holding you back from fulfilling your wildest dreams? What obstacles, real or imagined, are in your way? You have the tools to free yourself of them now. Cut through the perceived limitations. You are in charge of your thoughts. You alone have the power to transform your future. Your vulnerability is a crown of glory, an honest embrace of who you truly are and a stamp of resilience.

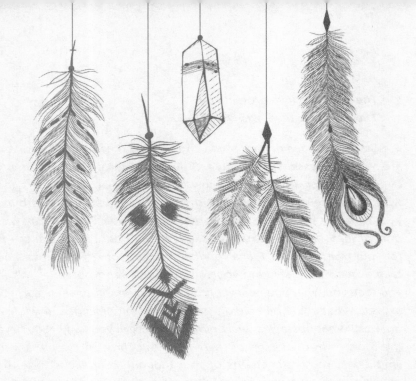

"*Caring for myself is not self-indulgence, it is self-preservation, and that is an act of political warfare.*"

- Audre Lorde-

feminist, womanist, and civil-rights activist

MOTIVATION MIX TRACK:
"CRANES IN THE SKY"
by Solange, *A Seat at the Table*

AFTERWORD

Beloved,

Harness your creative energy, follow your glow power, and navigate life from a place of soul connection. You are in partnership with a larger force. You have a compelling vision to carry through the vicissitudes of your journey. Create a lineage of your own. Don't wait for another day to go by before you pursue your vision to the fullest. Only you can create your blueprint for success. Everything is in divine progress. We are moving on a continuum, and there is no end point, but there is a beginning, and it is *you*. You are the beginning of a movement.

Breathe. Soften. Open. Stimulate your inner desire for knowledge, create space for what inspires you, move in spite of fear, and connect with your higher self to gain a clear vision of your true path. Nourish your spirit, sharpen your senses, and deepen your personal glow power. You have the courage to act on your intuition. You have the discernment and intuitive listening skills to know when you need to slow down and tap into the portal of self-renewal and practice self-care. By connecting with your magic, you create the strength to move through life's challenges with ease and clarity. You are powerful and limitless. Hold steadfast to the vision, trust the process, and lift your heart and keep your head held high to the sky.

Everything we experience is a part of us and becomes a part of our cosmic imprint. Women are storytellers filled with creative forces at work within. It's time to tell your story. There is intelligence at work within each of your cells, spinning life into existence. You were born a creatrix. Evoke your alchemical magic, ignite your passion and purpose, and embody the queen you were born to be.

Be present with your voice. Free it. Speak your truth and never again live in silence. Embrace that which makes you uniquely feminine; harness your power for the greatest good. If we can connect to that creative center—listening to it, feeding it, nurturing it—we can grow within ourselves something much bigger and offer it up to the world. Not leaning in, but rising up and standing tall—crowned. This is my ultimate wish for you. Nurture the seed growing within. Believe in the twinkling star that you are. Be your own disciple. Spread your stardust. Own it! Rise up, shine forth, and glow!

Love & Guidance,

Latham Thomas

"We are chemically connected to all molecules on Earth. And we are atomically connected to all atoms in the universe. We are not figuratively, but literally stardust."

– Neil deGrasse Tyson

ACKNOWLEDGMENTS

*G*iving thanks. All glory to God who worked through me to deliver this book.

Sometimes you sit down and place your hands on the keyboard, and the words flow fluidly through your fingers and write themselves. God goes off, and through you, channels medicine through your message that will heal when eyes lay upon your words. Other times, you sit down and start drafting . . . Well, I never allowed myself to just sit down and draft. I only wrote words that spun inside my core, and I would get up if I wasn't in the right state of being. I would move my body, do some breath work, take a walk, gaze at flowers, and come back when inspired and in the flow. Sometimes I didn't write for months at a time, but when I sat down, it always felt cathartic. The handling of language and the touch of every word is an opportunity to soften, open, and set free those whose eyes fall upon these pages. And I am thankful for the wisdom to do just that, to be intentional, so I could deliver this exact work as it is now to you.

This work was created over a period of time and there is a beautiful arc of growth that carries this book forward. I am ever thankful for the patience of my editor Lisa Cheng at Hay House for being a gentle yet firm guide and hands-on liaison in the final days of production. I am deeply grateful to the angel that is Shanna Milkey for stepping in and guiding me to organize my vision and being an incredible editor, and working on the book while in her final stretch of pregnancy. I am so grateful for the love and encouragement of my mother and father, Terry Carter and William Thomas, who have instilled in me a strong sense of self and who have always allowed me to be who I truly am. I want to acknowledge my beloved fiancé for giving me the space to go underground when I needed to write and being my greatest fan and supporter. Thank you, Fulano, my greatest joy and the inspiration for everything I do; Mama loves you. To my sister Nicole, I love you and your whimsical spirit; deep bow, my angel! Thank you to Granny for praying over me constantly and being a voice of optimism no matter what. Salute to Grandpa for always making me laugh. I am so blessed to have you both in my life.

I'm deeply moved by the support and guidance of friends who believe in me. Thank you to: Rachel Ash, Andrea Jackson, Saundra Parks, Alicia Keys, Opal Tometi, Knowledge Katti, Sarah Jones, India.Arie, June Ambrose, Sara Auster, Tiffany Dufu, Morin Oluwole, Caralene Robinson, Gigi Parris, Tai Beauchamp, De'Ara Balenger, Zac Posen, Molly Gochman, Kimberly Chandler, Dream Hampton, Sara Sophie Flicker, Elaine Welteroth, Rebecca Walker, Sarah Lewis, Tammy Brook, Lisa Price, Debra Lee, Thelma Golden, Jeanette Jenkins, Maya Watson, Tina Wells, Deirdre Maloney, Sandra Richards, Crystal McCrary, Shauna Neely, Shauna Mei, Ieesha Reed, Sharifa Murdock, Tricia and Antoinette Clarke, Maxie McCoy, Michelle Gadsden Williams, Nicole Ari Parker, Raquel Cepeda, Morgan Shara, Jessica Stark, Mara Brock Akil, Adrienne Bosh, Angela Simmons, Gabrielle Union, Jeanine Liburd, Terri Cole, Janete Rodas, Michele Promaulayko, Bozoma St. John, Terri Hines, Sheereen Russell, Tonya Lewis Lee, Tara Stiles, Amy Hanlon, Anita Kopacz, Agapi Stassinopoulos, Anna Kenney, Michelle Mitchum, Sonja Nuttall, Gianne Doherty, and Tracey Henry—I see you.

To all of the women who put their trust in me and allow me to support and witness them in birth—thank you. Each of you have impacted my life and we are forever bonded in birth. So much gratitude to my OWN family and to Ms. Oprah Winfrey for lifting me and my work. Thank you to my book agent Steve Harris, and to Michele Martin. To the incomparable Dawn Davis, who went above and beyond to help me navigate the editorial waters. Patty Gift, thank you for seeing a leader in me and taking a chance so many years ago and giving me the space to give rise to the book I was meant to write—it's finally here. Thank you to the Hay House matriarch Louise Hay for holding the space for all of your authors. I am so blessed and so thankful.

GLOW GLOSSARY

Altar — A sacred space designed to welcome spiritual energies into your space. It's an embodiment of your internal spiritual landscape and serves as a window to the Divine.

Beditation — A meditation practice conducted by lying down in bed or on the floor supported by pillows and props.

Body Scan — A meditative pathway to full presence, using awareness or mindfulness to awaken the whole body.

Confessions of Light — The opposite of a traditional confession. An opportunity to speak about the inspiration and acknowledge people who have made a beauty mark on your life.

Conscious Calendaring — Making an intentional effort to account for your whole being and self-care when planning your schedule by checking in internally, specifically around your monthly menses.

Creatrix — One who harnesses creative energy and transforms it into something manifest.

Crowned — Confident with head held high, standing firmly in your glow power on a pedestal you built for yourself.

Crystal — A pure solid substance that has an orderly repeating arrangement of atoms and molecules in the three spatial dimensions. Crystals like rose quartz, amethyst, citrine, agate, and tiger's eye are commonly used for energy healing.

Deep Listening — An act of fully present listening where one is still with awareness and tapped into the gravity of the moment. Giving attention. Listening beyond the sound.

Essential Oils — A potent natural oil typically obtained by distillation and having the characteristic fragrance of the plant from which it is extracted.

Feminine Edge — One's unique feminine magic that sets her apart from everyone else.

Flower Essences — Herbal infusions or decoctions made from the flowering part of the plant, which uniquely address the emotional and mental aspects of wellness.

Glow Foods — Whole plant-based foods, superfoods packed with antioxidants, minerals, and powerful nutrients that help combat inflammation, balance the hormonal system, keep insulin levels low, and promote healthy weight management.

Glow Guidance — Mentorship, cheerleading, and support to help guide you to the next level of excellence.

Glow Power — That innate creative force within all women—cosmic-creation vibration, that potent instinctual energy that awakens within us, plus fierce femininity.

Glow Time — A self-care practice rooted in slowing down, decompressing, and honoring one's needs—mental, physical, emotional, and spiritual. Checking out with the world around you to check in with yourself.

Glownership — Claiming ownership over a life of fulfillment that is your birthright. Owning your glow.

GPS (Glow Power System) — Your intuitive voice. Your God-given, internal compass, your built-in guidance and navigation, GPS.

Grounding — Anchoring oneself in the present moment. Also a form of therapeutic healing, where one spends time barefoot connecting with electromagnetic charge of the earth.

Growing Edge — Our most vulnerable blind spot, the area where we most need to grow.

Holding Space — To provide a container of safety, security, and an opportunity for a process of personal growth to unfold.

Intention — A deep desire, purpose, or focused objective carried out by the great organizing power of the universe. A compass that serves to keep us aligned with our goals, which are an extension of our intention.

Intuition — Your built-in GPS, Glow Power System, or internal guidance.

Invocation — Summoning forth energy through words or song.

Mala — A string of beads commonly used while reciting, chanting, or mentally repeating a mantra or prayer.

Mantra — Where mind and heart meet with the voice to make a sacred sound. We chant mantras to activate or evoke certain energy.

Meditation — Referring to a broad variety of mindfulness practices, including techniques designed to promote relaxation, build your internal energy or life force, and develop compassion, love, patience, generosity, and forgiveness. This practice helps us to induce modes of consciousness related to overall well-being.

Mindfulness — Paying attention intentionally. A mental state achieved by focusing one's awareness on the present moment, while calmly acknowledging and accepting one's feelings, thoughts, and bodily sensations, used as part of a therapeutic technique.

Moon Mapping — Attuning to and utilizing the lunar phases as a principal guide for your organizing aspects of your life, including career, romance, social, etc.

Moonifesting — To use the power of the lunar phases to bring your vision into fruition.

Portal — A pathway, gate, or doorway into a world

Ritual — A series of actions performed with intention that amplify the magic in everyday moments.

Sacred Anatomy — The matrix of feminine genitalia as well as reproductive organs and the erectile network responsible for female arousal and orgasm.

Seed Goal — A dense goal that we nurture through our intentions and actions.

Smudge Wand — A bundle of dried herbs, usually bound with string into a small bundle. These herbs are burned as part of a ritual or ceremony.

Triple Goddess — A trifecta symbol that represents the Maiden, Mother, and Crone as the waxing, full, and waning moon. It is also associated with wild feminine energy, mystery, and psychic abilities.

Wombifest — To hold space or create a container for what you most desire, drawing resources toward yourself and allowing the process of cultivation to unfold. Letting it happen, rather than *making* it happen.

Queendom — One's feminine energetic domain.

Queening — Reveling in your royalty, sanctity, and divinity.

RESOURCES

Astrology

My favorite resources for astrological tools, reflections, and wisdom.

- AstroStyle — astrostyle.com
- Cosmo Muse — cosmomuse.com
- My Path Astrology — mypathastrology.com
- Mystic Mamma — mysticmamma.com
- The Numinous — the-numinous.com

Beauty

My beauty must-haves and resources for clean, green, and holistic beauty that works!

- Art of Organics — artoforganics.com
- CAP Beauty — spa.capbeauty.com
- EcoDiva Beauty — ecodivabeauty.com
- Follain — shopfollain.com
- Fresh — fresh.com
- Good Medicine Beauty Lab — goodmedicinebeautylab.com
- Leahlani Skin Care — leahlaniskincare.com
- Naturopathica — naturopathica.com
- Palermo Body — palermobody.com
- Shiva Rose — shivarose.com
- Tammy Fender — tammyfender.com
- Tata Harper — tataharperskincare.com
- Vivrant Beauty — vivrantbeauty.com

Business and Entrepreneurship

For anyone on their own business journey or working toward entrepreneurship, you will love these spaces designed to help you thrive.

- Career Contessa — careercontessa.com
- Create & Cultivate — createcultivate.com
- Girlboss — girlboss.com
- Levo — levo.com
- Rising Tide Society — risingtidesociety.com
- WeWork — wework.com

Communities

These women-centric digital communities will spark inspiration and idea sharing.

- bSmart — bsmartguide.com
- Mogul — onmogul.com
- OKREAL — okreal.co
- Women For One — womenforone.com

Conferences

I believe in surrounding yourself with people who challenge your mind and help propel your growth. Here are some of the women-centric conferences that I think are worthy of your bucket list.

- BlogHer — blogher.com
- EmpowerHER — empowerherconference.com
- MAKERS — makers.com
- S.H.E. Summit — shesummit.com
- Well Summit — wellsummit.org
- What Women Want Conference — whatwomenwantconference.com
- Yellow Conference — yellowco.co

Décor and Home

I'm a huge fan of beautiful spaces, and these resources are excellent for decorating any space.

- ArtStar — artstar.com
- Artifact Uprising — artifactuprising.com
- Casper — casper.com

- Homepolish — homepolish.com
- Jonathan Adler — jonathanadler.com
- Lulu + Georgia — luluandgeorgia.com
- Minted — minted.com
- One Kings Lane — onekingslane.com
- Serena & Lily — serenaandlily.com
- twelvehome — twelvehomedesign.com

Fashion and Style

Your style statement should be reflective of who you are. Here are some of my favorite brands, shops, and e-retailers to style up your wardrobe.

- Anthropologie — anthropologie.com
- BANDIER — bandier.com
- Basic Terrain — basicterrain.com
- eberjey — eberjey.com
- J.Crew — jcrew.com
- Lou & Grey — louandgrey.com
- LoveShackFancy — loveshackfancy.com
- Mara Hoffman — marahoffman.com
- NET-A-PORTER — net-a-porter.com
- Rebecca Minkoff — rebeccaminkoff.com
- Zac Posen — zacposen.com
- Zuvaa — zuvaa.com

Femme Care

For all of your feminine needs—whether self-pleasure, menses, or protection—I've got you covered.

- Elvie — elvie.com
- genneve — genneve.com
- Intimina — intimina.com
- JimmyJane — jimmyjane.com
- Kali — kaliboxes.com
- LOLA — mylola.com
- Negative Underwear — negativeunderwear.com
- Sustain Natural — sustainnatural.com
- THINX — shethinx.com

Inspiration

These sites inspire lifestyle goals; just bookmark them!

- 21Ninety — 21ninety.com
- *Belong Magazine* — belong-mag.com
- Glitter Guide — glitterguide.com
- goop — goop.com
- Grit & Virtue — gritandvirtue.com
- Kinfolk — kinfolk.com
- SuperSoul — supersoul.tv
- Thrive Global — thriveglobal.com

Magazines and Media

These magazines are reframing beauty, self-care, and the way women celebrate themselves.

- *CRWNMAG* — crwnmag.com
- *Darling Magazine* — darlingmagazine.org
- *HANNAH* magazine — hannahmag.com
- Paper Monday — papermonday.com
- *Saint Heron* — saintheron.com
- *Thoughtfully Magazine* — thoughtfullymag.com

Meditation and Mindfulness

These resources have everything you need to deepen your meditation and mindfulness practice.

- Headspace — headspace.com
- Inscape — inscape.life
- Mindful — mindful.org
- MNDFL — mndflmeditation.com
- Modern ŌM — modernom.co
- SAMAYA — samaya.life
- *Tricycle* magazine — tricycle.org
- Unplug Meditation — unplugmeditation.com

Nutrition

You are what you consume, and below you will find some of my favorite things to consume for ultimate well-being.

- Anima Mundi Herbals — animamundiherbals.com
- Beaming — livebeaming.com
- Herbalore NYC — herbalorenyc.com
- Moon Juice — moonjuiceshop.com
- Movita Organics — movitaorganics.com
- Ritual — ritual.com
- Sakara Life — sakara.com
- TYME Fast Food — tymefood.com

Ritual and Spirituality

These resources will help you adorn your surroundings and outfit your life with the ritual affects that resonate with your personal style.

- ABC Carpet & Home — abchome.com
- Advisory Board Crystals — advisoryboardcrystals.com
- Incausa — incausa.co
- Lotus Wei — lotuswei.com
- Modern Women — modernwomen.bigcartel.com
- Otherwild — otherwild.com
- Species by the Thousands — speciesbythethousands.com
- Tiny Devotions — lovetinydevotions.com
- The Wild Unknown — thewildunknown.com

Self-Care

Self-care is an integral part of your journey to the glow. Here are some resources that can help you slow down, tune inward, and honor your mental, emotional, and physical need for well-being.

- Carol's Daughter — carolsdaughter.com
- Fat and the Moon — fatandthemoon.com
- Mama Glow — mamaglow.com
- *Organic Spa Magazine* — organicspamagazine.com
- Pursoma — pursomalife.com
- Saje Natural Wellness — saje.com
- Sparitual — sparitual.com

- TalkSpace — talkspace.com
- The Local Rose — thelocalrose.com
- Queen Afua Wellness Center — queenafua.com

Travel and Wanderlust

When it's time to take a trip, here is where I go for travel inspiration:

- AFAR — afar.com
- *Boat Magazine* — boat-mag.com
- *Condé Nast Traveler* — cntraveler.com
- FP Escapes — freepeople.com/fpescapes
- Pravassa — pravassa.com
- Travel Noire — travelnoire.com

Yoga

If you need a really awesome travel mat or the cutest yoga pants the world has to offer, you'll find what you need in this list:

- *Aligned Magazine* — alignedmag.com
- Carbon38 — carbon38.com
- La Vie Boheme Yoga — laviebohemeyoga.com
- Manduka Yoga — manduka.com
- Wanderlust — wanderlust.com
- Yoga Design Lab — yogadesignlab.com

ABOUT THE AUTHOR

*L*ATHAM THOMAS, aka Glow Maven, is a celebrity wellness/ lifestyle maven and birth doula who transforms not only how women give birth to their babies, but how they give rise to the best version of themselves. Named one of Oprah Winfrey's Super Soul 100, an enlightened group of leaders elevating humanity with their work, Latham is helping women embrace optimal wellness and spiritual growth as a pathway to empowerment. She is the founder of Mama Glow (MamaGlow.com), a lifestyle brand and highly regarded website offering inspiration, education, and holistic services for expectant and new mamas. A graduate of Columbia University and The Institute for Integrative Nutrition, Latham formerly served on the advisory board of Yahoo! Health and currently she serves on the TUFTS University Nutrition Council. Latham is the best-selling author of *Mama Glow: A Hip Guide to Your Fabulous Abundant Pregnancy*, a go-to wellness guide for expecting mothers endorsed by Dr. Christiane Northrup, Dr. Mark Hyman, Christy Turlington Burns, Dr. Frank Lipman, and more.

Having cultivated her wellness practice for over nearly a decade, she has served as a doula and lifestyle guru for such celebrity clients as Alicia Keys, Rebecca Minkoff, Tamera Mowry, and Venus and Serena Williams. A self-proclaimed *ritualista*, Latham believes in turning the ordinary routines of everyday life into sacred moments. Whether involved in travel, dining, self-care, style, fitness, mindfulness, or well-being, Latham is guided by inspiration and celebrates moments of magic in the mundane.

Latham is leading a revolution in radical self-care by helping women everywhere to reclaim their queendom and teaching them to "mother themselves first." She was named one of the "Top 100 Women to Watch in Wellness" by mindbodygreen. A single mom residing in NYC, she is the proud mother of DJ prodigy and entrepreneur DJ Fulano. Latham has been featured in a variety of media outlets, including *Vogue*, *SELF*, Fast Company, *Wall Street Journal Magazine*, *E! News*, *Essence*, Fit Pregnancy, My Domaine, DuJour, *Forbes*, BET Networks, *The Dr. Oz Show*, Centric, *Good Day New York*, and *Inside Edition*.

HAY HOUSE TITLES OF RELATED INTEREST

YOU CAN HEAL YOUR LIFE, the movie,
starring Louise Hay & Friends
(available as a 1-DVD program, an expanded 2-DVD set, and an online streaming video)
Learn more at www.hayhouse.com/louise-movie

THE SHIFT, the movie,
starring Dr. Wayne W. Dyer
(available as a 1-DVD program, an expanded 2-DVD set, and an online streaming video)
Learn more at www.hayhouse.com/the-shift-movie

YOU ARE AMAZING: A Help-Yourself Guide for Trusting Your Vibes + Reclaiming Your Magic,
by Sonia & Sabrina Choquette-Tully

THE HEART OF AROMATHERAPY:
An Easy-to-Use Guide for Essential Oils,
by Andrea Butje

STRALA YOGA:
Be Strong, Focused & Ridiculously Happy from the Inside Out,
by Tara Stiles

All of the above are available at your local bookstore,
or may be ordered by contacting Hay House (see next page).

We hope you enjoyed this Hay House book. If you'd like to receive our online catalog featuring additional information on Hay House books and products, or if you'd like to find out more about the Hay Foundation, please contact:

Hay House, Inc., P.O. Box 5100, Carlsbad, CA 92018-5100
(760) 431-7695 or (800) 654-5126
(760) 431-6948 (fax) or (800) 650-5115 (fax)
www.hayhouse.com® • www.hayfoundation.org

Published in Australia by: Hay House Australia Pty. Ltd.,
18/36 Ralph St., Alexandria NSW 2015
Phone: 612-9669-4299 • *Fax:* 612-9669-4144
www.hayhouse.com.au

Published in the United Kingdom by: Hay House UK, Ltd.,
The Sixth Floor, Watson House, 54 Baker Street, London W1U 7BU
Phone: +44 (0)20 3927 7290 • *Fax:* +44 (0)20 3927 7291
www.hayhouse.co.uk

Published in India by: Hay House Publishers India,
Muskaan Complex, Plot No. 3, B-2, Vasant Kunj, New Delhi 110 070
Phone: 91-11-4176-1620 • *Fax:* 91-11-4176-1630
www.hayhouse.co.in

Access New Knowledge.
Anytime. Anywhere.

Learn and evolve at your own pace
with the world's leading experts.

www.hayhouseU.com

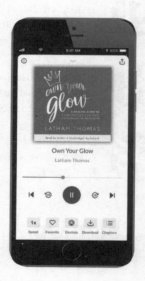